Jumptown

Jumptown
The Golden Years of Portland Jazz, 1942-1957

BY ROBERT DIETSCHE

Oregon State University Press
Corvallis

Library of Congress Cataloging-in-Publication Data

Dietsche, Robert.

 Jumptown : the golden years of Portland jazz, 1942-1957 / Robert Dietsche ; foreword by James L. Swenson ; afterword by Lynn A. Darroch.

     p. cm.

 Includes bibliographical references, discography, and index.

 ISBN-10: 0-87071-114-8 (alk. paper)

 ISBN-13: 978-0-87071-114-5 (alk. paper)

 1. Jazz--Oregon--Portland--History and criticism. 2. Jazz musicians--Oregon--Portland. 3. Nightclubs--Oregon--Portland. I. Title.

 ML3508.8.P6D53 2005

 781.65'09795'49--dc22

                          2005006366

♾ This paper meets the requirements of ANSI/NISO Z39.48-1992 (Permanence of Paper).

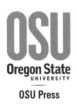
OSU
Oregon State
UNIVERSITY
OSU Press

Oregon State University Press
121 The Valley Library
Corvallis OR 97331
541-737-3166 • fax 541-737-3170
www.osupress.oregonstate.edu

DEDICATION

For J. D. D.
and the Earth Angel

Table of Contents

The purpose of this book is to shed light on a time and a place that have been written out of Portland history and jazz history in general. Much of the story takes place in an urban Black community with its own way of doing things, a community most people today do not know existed, but one that Jack Kerouac, author of *On the Road,* would have found irresistible. Another purpose is to pay respect to the musicians and the dancers, to the jazz educators and jazz journalists, to the jazz jockeys who molded tastes on the radio, and the tape jockeys who spent their nights in the back row of some smoky cafe watching a reel-to-reel recorder turn. This book is for the promoters, the ballroom managers, and the club owners, and all the patrons who made 1942 to 1957 the golden years of Portland jazz. What follows is a guided tour of the most talked about jazz spots and the jazz people who inhabited them.

Foreword

When most people think of the origins of jazz, Portland, Oregon, is not the first place that comes to mind. And yet, for a golden decade following World War II, the coincidence of a port city, a busy railroad, and a bustling shipbuilding industry caused a confluence of musical interest and talent rarely rivaled on the West Coast. It was a confluence whose effects last to this day.

Duke Ellington, Gene Krupa, Ella Fitzgerald, Charlie Parker, Benny Goodman, Coleman Hawkins, Thelonious Monk—many of the world's emerging jazz giants loved to play Portland and trade chops with up and coming local talent.

"Action central was Williams Avenue, an entertainment strip lined with hot spots where you could find jazz twenty-four hours a day," writes Bob Dietsche. "You could stand in the middle of the Avenue (where the Blazers play basketball today) and look up Williams past the chili parlors, past the barbecue joints, the beauty salons, all the way to Broadway, and see hundreds of people dressed up as if they were going to a fashion show. It could be four in the morning. It didn't matter; this was one of those 'streets that never slept.' "

This book for the first time collects hundreds of disparate pieces of local jazz history—photographs, news clips, reviews, personal recollections, maps, handbills—to reconstruct the era of early jazz in Portland. From a Depression-era WPA marching band to a roly-poly music teacher named Wally Hanna, this book shows jazz fans how the roots of jazz grew into a music that has influenced musicians in Portland today.

Who were the pioneers that brought jazz to Oregon? How did Portland become such a jazz hot spot? What role did the Kaiser shipyards play? How does the Bonneville Dam figure in? What about all those "after-hours speakeasies?" This book identifies and profiles some fifty players, band leaders, music teachers, critics, fans, and promoters, who spread the word in Oregon about America's "new music" and who encouraged or introduced jazz here. It brings forward the sounds and techniques of those early players. It shines a light on the clubs and dance halls that were the hot spots.

Take a walk up the Avenue from the hot sounds of the Dude Ranch (until recently a plastics store) over to the Acme. Pop into McClendon's Rhythm Room, then to the Frat Hall. Let's stop over at McElroy's, the Coop, and Paul's Paradise. We could take in the big bands at Jantzen Beach. *Jumptown* takes us into the clubs that were the main venues of the driving jazz scene in the 1940s and 1950s. From supper club to speakeasy, it captures the ambiance, the personalities, the stories of this rip-roaring period of Portland's past. It celebrates and at the same time preserves a part of our cultural past which has greatly influenced our cultural present.

Jim Swenson

Jim Swenson is an independent film director in Portland

Acknowledgments

This book is indebted to Nick Ceroli, Fred Lutz, Lee "One Putt" Raymond, and Bernie Kehoe for turning my ears in the right direction. Also to George L. Beardsly for giving me his 1925 thesaurus. And thanks to Ray Krebsbach at Eastern Washington University for making sense out of English grammar; to Herb Nelson at Oregon State University for making English Lit swing; to University of Oregon's Kester Svenson for unlocking the mysteries of *Paradise Lost*; and David Tyack at Reed College who could teach calculus to cavemen.

I am grateful to Gene Confer for ten years of music appreciation.

Credit should go to my research sources: *The People's Observer, The Northwest Enterprise*, Dan Morgenstern and the Institute of Jazz Studies, *The Oregonian, The Oregon Journal*, the Oregon Historical Society, and the Multnomah County Library.

This book owes plenty to the Cogan brothers, Garth Miller, and Eric Duckstad for the use of their vast libraries of jazz.

I am thankful for the inspiration I got from jazz books by Gunther Schuller, Leroy Ostransky, Paul de Barros, Robert Gordon, Ted Gioia, and historian Frederick Lewis Allen.

For their generous supply of photos, I thank Ted Hallock, Margaret Havlicek, Virginia Black, Bernice Slaughter, the Amato family, Joanne Hasbrouck, James Benton, the McClendon family, Phil Hunt, Cleve Williams, George Reinmiller, and Julie James, Documart's copy queen.

A huge salute goes out to recording engineers Bob Redfern and Bob Thompson for fifty years of Portland jazz on tape.

For their editorial contribution and encouragement, thanks to Marianne Keddington-Lang, Eve Goodman, Ellen Teicher, and Penny Harrison. And thanks to Margaret Knispel, Bob Crowley, and Pat Joy for their confidence in my ability.

To John Henley, Phil Wikelund, Mark Christensen, and Dave Kelly, thanks for some very wise advice.

My appreciation to Nate Nickerson, Bob Coleman, Katherine Bogle, and the Unthank family for their historical perspectives.

And I owe much to the Jumptown Seven, who tried to make a CD-ROM out of this book and would have succeeded except for the financial repercussions of 9/11. They are Leslie Rosenberg, Dick Bogle, Ted Hallock, Ron Weber, Jim Swenson, Garth Miller, and ace photographer Bob Trowbridge, who spent countless hours developing and improving the photos for this book.

I was lucky to have such thorough researchers as Gloria Myers Horowitz, Ron Weber, Neville Eschen, Garth Miller, Leslie Rosenberg, and Suzanne Hanchett. And a big hug to Joyce Atkins for the use of her high-speed stenography machine.

My lasting appreciation to Mary Elizabeth Braun for her belief in *Jumptown* and for guiding me through the necessary steps toward publication. Kudos also go out to the tasty cover design, and to copy editor Jo Alexander, who can make an apprentice look like a pro.

And finally to my wife, Susan, without whom this book would not have been written.

Introduction

Without Franklin Delano Roosevelt, two congressmen, and a man from Salem, Oregon, the story of jazz in Portland would be completely different. It must have been Gunther Schuller who said that region and accident are the two most powerful factors in the development of jazz. You can double that for Portland. If it were not for the completion of Bonneville Dam in 1937, the golden decade of jazz and the flowering of Williams Avenue would never have happened. It was the cheap power produced by this engineering marvel on the Columbia that attracted Kaiser shipyards and other defense industries during World War II. Had it not been for the lobbying power and the indefatigable perseverance of future Governor Charles Martin and Senator Charles McNary, the Bonneville Dam would not have been built in time for World War II. The grand migration of Black workers from the South and the music they brought with them would not have arrived.

FDR, whose idea for the dam was part of his 1932 candidacy, had put it on the back burner and was postponing the construction in favor of spending more money on Grand Coulee Dam. McNary and Martin, fearing that it would be put on hold indefinitely, raced to Washington in an effort to change FDR's mind. They were told that the President was too busy to see them because he was getting ready for an extended vacation. They remained in the waiting room with dozens of other people who urgently wanted a last-minute audience with the President. Enter an old friend from Salem, Oregon, now FDR's personal secretary, Marvin McIntire. When he came over to greet them, they told him of their dilemma and within minutes he had arranged a meeting with the President. Then Martin went to work. In a flash of brilliant thinking he told the President that he would be following in the footsteps of Thomas Jefferson. "By this act you are sending out a new Lewis and Clark Expedition to rediscover the Pacific Northwest. This part of the country has been held back by lack of power. By this act you are harnessing the Columbia River and giving us an unlimited supply of the cheapest power in the country. And by doing that you will rebuild the Northwest."[1] The inspired rhetoric worked and FDR gave them the 36 million dollars they needed for the Corps of Engineers to begin immediately. That was September 1933.

Who's Who in Jumptown

Amadee, Leo: the beginning of bop piano in Portland

Amato, Sam: drummer, ballroom operator, and promoter

Anderson, Don: durable band leader, teacher, classically trained pianist with a flair for jazz

Anderson, Quen: trombonist, expert arranger, and composer

Ballou, Monte: banjo-strumming, indomitable leader of the Castle Jazz Band

Beach, Ed: noted jazz broadcaster, pianist, historian

Benton, James: drummer, blues singer, and Avenue historian

Black, Warren: harmonically advanced bassist and electric guitarist, an instrument he brought to the forefront in Portland

Bogle, Dick: former city commissioner and still-active jazz writer, photographer, and disc jockey

Bracken, Warren: pianist, singer, and leader of the Avenue's young at bop

Bradford, Bobby: Cleve Williams's alter ego and for forty years the leading light of bebop trumpet in Portland

Bridges, Walter: energetic headmaster of Portland's most famous big band workshop

Brown, Braley: saxophonist, bassist, poet, and life of the jam session

Chaney, Art: veteran saxophonist and historian

Confer, Gene: Portland's piano patriarch

Day, Basie: Leroy Vinnegar-type bassist with big beat

Duke, Stanton: pioneer promoter of Black big bands

Garret, Charlie: Kansas City-born founder of Madrona Records and the Ballot Box with the business IQ of a Louis Rukeyser

Geller, Lorraine Walsh: Rose City's most highly acclaimed jazz pianist

Hale, Teddy: Gene Krupa in taps

Hallock, Ted: former state senator, drummer, bandleader, disc jockey, and *Down Beat* correspondent whose articles put Portland on the jazz map

The Hamiltones: forty years of swing

Hanna, Wally: Vancouver High School's Mr. Holland

Heider, Wally: Sheridan, Oregon's saxophonist, band leader, and world-famous recording engineer

Henson, Julian: the best unknown pianist in town

Hilliard, William: publisher of *Portland Challenger*, former editor of *The Oregonian*, prime witness to events on the Avenue

Hing, Kenny: tenor saxophonist and only Portlander to win a membership in the Count Basie band

Hood, Bill: One of the unknown giants of the baritone sax

Hood, Ernie: guitarist, zitherist, composer, graphic artist, broadcaster, and Portland's first jazz historian

Horn, Ray: dulcet-toned disc jockey, competitive swing dancer, drummer, and man about jazz for over half a century

Jackson, Roy: River City's Wardell Gray

Jacquet, Illinois: Lionel Hampton-associated saxophonist with an enormous influence on the Avenue

Johnson, Dink: Portland's most distinguished jazz resident

Johnson, Tom: The godfather in every sense of the word

Keller, Freddie: former trombonist with Jack Teagarden and dance-band leader

Killian, Al: leader of the great quintet of 1947, starring Wardell Gray and Sonny Criss, appearing nightly on the Avenue

Kinch, Don: superb New Orleans-style cornetist and band leader

Knight, Dick: tenor saxophonist with a sound and swing of a ballroom slugger

Lawson, George: alto saxophonist and the Avenue's most likely to succeed

Levitt, Rod: trombonist, arranger, composer, and leader of the best little big band in the 1960s

McAnulty, Bob, and Taylor, Sammy: jazz broadcasting à la mode

McClendon, Bill: night-club owner, pianist, newspaper columnist, civil rights activist, and educator

McElroy, Cole ("Pop"): ballroom owner, band leader, and early integrationist

Moore, Phil: piano prodigy, co-inventor of the block chord piano style, arranger, and world-famous vocal coach

Pierre, Al: pianist and leader of Portland's most successful Black band of the 1930s

Porter, Sid: Portland's gentle giant of jazz piano

Rockey, Lee: modern drumming in Portland starts here

Rosenlund, Ralph: first major-league jazz saxophonist in Portland

Severinsen, Carl ("Doc"): poll-winning trumpeter and former leader of the Johnny Carson Tonight Show orchestra

Slaughter, Ed: pool-hall owner, historian, and honorary mayor of Williams Avenue

Spurgeon, Ray: lead altoist and the Woody Hite band's de facto leader

Thomas, Carl: Portland's original bebopper

Todd, Tommy: brilliant, enigmatic arranger, pianist for Benny Goodman, Tommy Dorsey, Harry James, and many other name bands of the forties

Turner, Burt: the Avenue's Music Man and jack of all instruments

Weathers, Roscoe: fireball alto saxophonist on loan from the Emerald City

Wendeborn, John: ex-trombonist, *The Oregonian* columnist, and jazz promoter since 1953

Wied, Eddie: a name synonymous with jazz piano in Portland

Williams, Clarence: vocalist, guitarist, and Portland's Prince of the Blues

Williams, Cleve: Portland's King of the Blues trombone

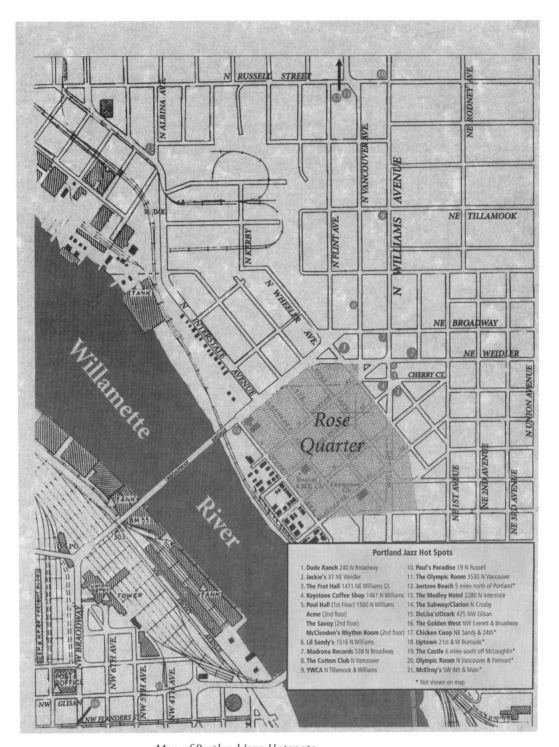

Portland Jazz Hot Spots

1. **Dude Ranch** 240 N Broadway
2. **Jackie's** 37 NE Weidler
3. **The Frat Hall** 1471 NE Williams Ct.
4. **Keystone Coffee Shop** 1461 N Williams
5. **Pool Hall** (1st Floor) 1500 N Williams
    Acme (2nd floor)
    The Savoy (2nd floor)
    McClendon's Rhythm Room (2nd floor)
6. **Lil Sandy's** 1516 N Williams
7. **Madrona Records** 538 N Broadway
8. **The Cotton Club** N Vancouver
9. **YWCA** N Tillamook & Williams
10. **Paul's Paradise** 19 N Russell
11. **The Olympic Room** 3530 N Vancouver
12. **Jantzen Beach** 5 miles north of Portland*
13. **The Medley Hotel** 2280 N Interstate
14. **The Subway/Clarion** N Crosby
15. **DeLisa's/Ozark** 425 NW Glisan
16. **The Golden West** NW Everett & Broadway
17. **Chicken Coop** NE Sandy & 24th*
18. **Uptown** 21st & W Burnside*
19. **The Castle** 6 miles south off McLoughlin*
20. **Olympic Room** N Vancouver & Fremont*
21. **McElroy's** SW 4th & Main*

* Not shown on map

Map of Portland Jazz Hotspots

CHAPTER 1

The Dude Ranch: Where Jump Was a Noun

Inland seaports with good railroads make for great jazz, especially during wartime, when there is an acceleration of fresh ideas and fashions from the thousands of servicemen and defense workers arriving.[1] Toledo, Ohio, Buffalo, New York, and Portland, Oregon, are good examples. So it is no surprise that Portland's golden years of jazz began just as World War II was ending.

During the war, tens of thousands of people, many of them Black and from Texas, had come to Portland to work in the Kaiser shipyards and other related areas of defense. When the war was over, most of the Blacks settled in an area that ran from the river to Northeast Fremont and east from North Interstate to Union Avenue, now called Martin Luther King Boulevard.[2] Part of this Little Harlem was set aside by city hall as a kind of tenderloin district and was operated by a Black vice lord named Tom Johnson. It used to be the cheapest land in town; now it's among the most expensive.

Action central was Williams Avenue, an entertainment strip lined with hot spots where you could find jazz twenty-four hours a day. What is now the Rose Quarter used to have a lot of other names. Any cabby worth his fare in those days would have known that Black Broadway, the other side, colored town, all meant the same thing: the Avenue,

namely Williams Avenue. Fifty years ago you could stand in the middle of the Avenue (where the Blazers play basketball today) and look up Williams past the chili parlors, past the barbecue joints, the beauty salons, all the way to Broadway, and see hundreds of people dressed up as if they were going to a fashion show. It could be four in the morning. It didn't matter; this was one of those "streets that never slept."[3]

And what were all these people looking for? Jazz mostly. There must have been more than ten clubs in as many blocks, not counting the ones in the surrounding area. There was the Frat Hall, home of Don Anderson, Sid Porter, Julian Henson, Al Pierre, and other pioneers of Portland jazz, where building inspectors were called in the morning after Ernie Fields rocked the foundation with his version of "T-town Blues." Across the street was the Savoy, where one night Wardell Gray blew twenty choruses of "Blue Lou" without once repeating himself. Down the street was Lil' Sandy's, where T-Bone Walker and Clarence Williams liked to play. Around the corner was Jackie's, where Leo Amadee showed the highly acclaimed Lorraine Walsh Geller how to play bebop piano. Near the corner of Williams and Russell was Paul's Paradise, where Seattle's Jabbo Ward and Billy Tolles would battle Portland's Roy Jackson in an all-out "cutting session."[4]

It is all gone now. Bulldozed away to make room for freeways and other manifestations of urban renewal, like some kind of Jazz Pompeii. All, that is, except for the Dude Ranch, that triangle-shaped building on the pie-shaped block that divides Weidler from North Broadway, about three hundred yards northwest of the Memorial Coliseum.

There never was and there never will be anything quite like the Dude Ranch. It was the Cotton Club, the Apollo Theater, Las Vegas, the Wild West rolled into one. It was the shooting star in the history of Portland jazz, a meteor bursting with an array of the best Black and Tan entertainment this town has ever seen: strippers, then called shake dancers, ventriloquists, comics, jugglers, torch singers, world-renowned tap dancers like Teddy Hale, and of course the very best of jazz.[5] What a jazz buff wouldn't give for a tape recorder and a front-row table the night Louis Armstrong dropped in from his dance date at Jantzen Beach. Or when Charlie Barnet sat in with the Banjoski house band or that August night just a couple of weeks after the end of World War II when Lucky Thompson and most of the Basie band showed up.[6]

In July of 1945, the Dude Ranch, with its tap-dancing MC and its celebrity clientele, was the hottest Black and Tan supper club west of Chicago. Less than a year later, the doors were locked. Some people downtown thought it was a public nuisance. Billie Holiday, Nat King Cole, and a host of other all-stars had to be canceled.

Built to be a hazelnut ice cream factory in 1908, it became a speakeasy in the 1920s. Until recently it was called Multi-Craft Plastics. Instead of dining, dancing, and gambling, it was plastics: residential, commercial, and industrial. The outside hadn't changed much since the days of the Dude. The inside had, and only an opening in the newly arranged false ceiling revealed the elaborately carved ceiling that once overlooked an even more elaborate dance floor.[7] The floor was mirrored and slippery and led to an elevated bandstand banked by rows of tables. Above and to the rear was an imposing balcony, and that is where you had dinner.

Photographers were everywhere. Folded cards in the middle of each table read, "You ain't nothing till you've had your photo taken at the Dude Ranch." Nod your head at the wrong time and you might find your face on the cover of matchbooks, calendars, or in *Let's Go*, Portland's main entertainment guide.

There were hatcheck girls, cigarette girls, and cowgirl waitresses dressed to look like Dale Evans, cardboard six-shooters snug in their holsters. Huge hand-painted murals of Black cowboys lassoing Texas longhorns covered the walls.[8]

Pat Patterson, the first Black ever to play basketball at the University of Oregon, owned and managed the Ranch with his pal Sherman "Cowboy" Pickett. They might have been inspired by a 1938 *Life* magazine article featuring heavyweight boxing champion Joe Louis learning to ride a horse at an all-Black dude ranch in Victorville, California.[9]

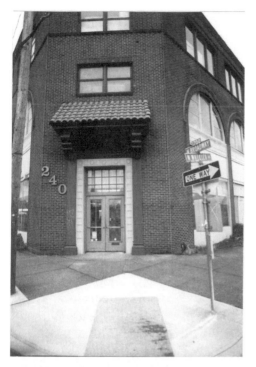

The Dude Ranch in 2005 (courtesy of Bob Trowbridge)

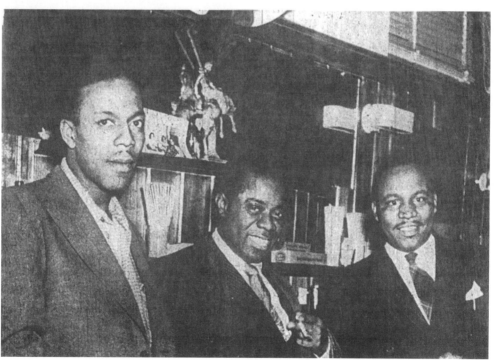

Pat Patterson, Louis Armstrong, and Sherman Pickett at the Dude Ranch (courtesy of Bernice Slaughter)

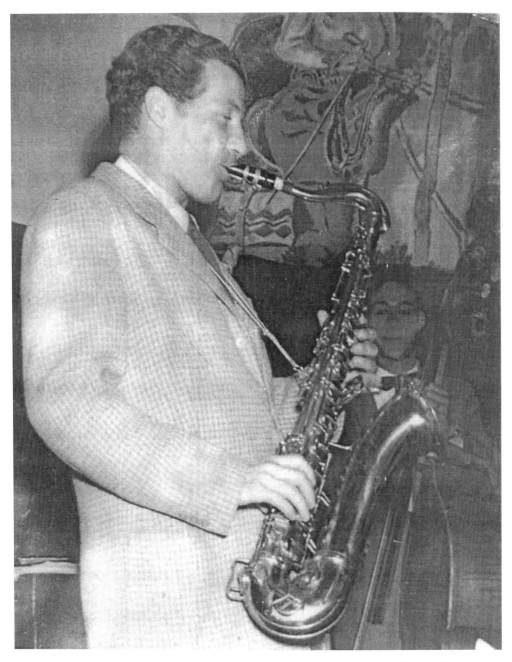

Charlie Barnet at the Dude Ranch (courtesy of McClendon family)

Louis was the Michael Jordan of 1945, maybe even bigger. "If you wanna know, watch Joe" was the forties version of "Be like Mike."

The Ranch was packed like every other place in this postwar boom town. Thousands of servicemen were passing through, home from the islands of the Pacific and crazy for entertainment. The money was easy; the housing was impossible. All-night movie theaters were converted into sleeping lodges; restaurants were telling people to stay home.[10] Portland, once thought to be the wallflower of the West Coast, had become a twenty-four-hour three-shift transport city going about 78 rpm. The fast- and free-spending crowd at the Dude Ranch was a reflection of that.

Among the well-dressed shipbuilders, maids, and Pullman porters were Bugsy Siegel-like characters in sharkskin suits and broad Panama hats in from St. Louis for a friendly game of cards or dice. One of them was Alligator Jack. There were pin-striped politicians with neon ties, Hollywood celebrities, and glamour queens in jungle-red nail polish and leopard coats.[11] There were feathered call girls and pimps in fake alligator shoes; zoot-suited hipsters and sidemen from Jantzen Beach looking to get the "taste of Guy Lombardo out of their mouths." Nobel Peace Prize candidates and petty thieves, Peggy Lee's "Big Spender" and Norman Mailer's *White Negro*. Racially mixed party people who couldn't care less that what they were doing was on the cutting edge of integration in the city that had been called the most segregated north of the Mason-Dixon line.

On Halloween of 1945, the crowd at the Ranch wouldn't let Joe Crane, Big Dave Henderson, and the rest of the Frantic Five off the stage. After their one-hour rendition of "St. Louis Blues," their loyal fans were yelling for one more encore.[12] But even that wouldn't compare with what happened on December 5 of that year, a date still talked about. That is when Norman Granz brought in the maiden voyage of Jazz at the Philharmonic, a traveling jam session named after its place of origin.

Granz, "the P. T. Barnum of jazz," was the first one to come up with the idea of putting the world's greatest jazz musicians on the road. He thus paved the way for all festivals to come, from Newport to Monterey to Mt. Hood. Even the recent success of the Portland Jazz Festival owes something to Norman Granz. He literally put jazz on the map, doing for the art form what Jack Kramer did for the game of tennis. Like Kramer, he took the best players in the world on a tour of the bigger cities in the U.S. They played mostly in theaters and town halls so that everyone, no matter what age, could attend. Then Granz decided to produce record albums recorded at various locations on the tours. He was one of the first to appreciate the value of liner notes and cover art and hired illustrator David Stone Martin to do all his albums.

In the forties, fifties, and sixties, thousands of people heard their first jazz at one of Granz's Philharmonic concerts.

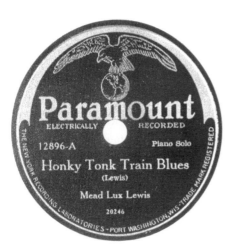

NORMAN GRANZ *presents . . .*

JAZZ at the PHILHARMONIC

It's gotten to the point where jazz is being called Art (and see that you spell that with a capital A, Jack) and the critical boys have picked it up, applied nice, big descriptive words about it, and before you know it, a jam session becomes a jazz concert, if you know what I mean. Or, as they sometimes like to put it, jazz is a folk music with its "roots sunk deep in the people." Actually, though, jazz, apart from its rhythm, and exciting improvisational qualities, is the one kind of a thing which, more than anything else, brings people together as spectators and participants with a complete disregard for race, color, or creed, and that, Jack, is more important than anything else that may be said of it as an "Art."

FIRST SET

DENZIL BEST—drums   COLEMAN HAWKINS—tenor sax
AL McKIBBON—bass   ROY ELDRIDGE—trumpet
THELONIOUS MONK—piano   LUCKY THOMPSON—tenor sax

Take Ten

* * *

SECOND SET

MEADE LUX LEWIS

* * *

THIRD SET

COLEMAN HAWKINS—tenor sax
THELONIOUS MONK—piano
DENZIL BEST—drums   AL McKIBBON—bass

Take Another Break

* * *

FOURTH SET

HELEN HUMES—vocal
DENZIL BEST—drums   COLEMAN HAWKINS—tenor sax
AL McKIBBON—bass   ROY ELDRIDGE—trumpet
THELONIOUS MONK—piano   LUCKY THOMPSON—tenor sax

*

NORMAN GRANZ—*Master of Ceremonies*

(Courtesy of Ted Hallock)

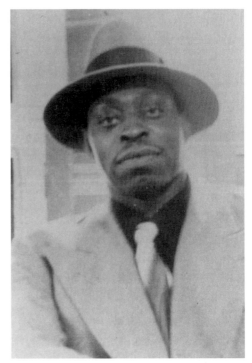

Alligator Jack (courtesy of Bob Williams)

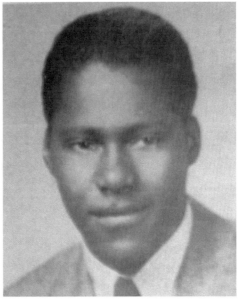

*Floyd Standifer at Gresham High School
(courtesy of Bob Trowbridge)*

But his most important contribution was in civil rights. Granz demanded a policy of equal rights be afforded each member of his integrated dream team. Any attempt to deny or compromise his accommodations was met with a firm cancellation.[13]

Granz brought some of the biggest names in jazz to the Dude Ranch on that December evening, including Roy Eldridge, Coleman Hawkins, and the then unknown Picasso of modern jazz, Thelonious Monk. Bill McClendon, writing in his own *People's Observer*, put it this way: "Never before in the history of the Northwest has there been as much jazz music played per square minute by any group." Eldridge "blew beyond the realm of imagination." Lucky Thompson was "intoxicating," Coleman Hawkins "incomparable."[14] Yet to McClendon they were just the under-card to the main event, Meade Lux Lewis, the Buddy Rich of boogie-woogie piano, who had the audience standing up, dancing in place.

Sitting at a table that night was Floyd Standifer, an eighteen-year-old trumpeter and future sideman of Quincy Jones. Standifer turned out to be one of the better trumpet players on the West Coast. That night he sat transfixed by the bizarre chords and extraterrestrial mannerisms of Monk. Chords that had Roy Eldridge grimacing and others laughing. "Here was this odd-looking guy who was making this room laugh. I learned about Monk from a magazine. I hitchhiked in from Gresham, where I was going to school and playing in a band. It took me a while to realize that what I first thought were mistakes and missing

notes were right according to what he was trying to do. He was getting a sound and energy out of the piano that couldn't be heard any other way," Standifer recalled.[15]

Before moving to Gresham, Floyd Standifer had spent the years 1936 to 1941 on Williams Avenue, where his father was a Methodist minister. One of the elder Standifer's duties was to hire a bandmaster as part of Franklin Delano Roosevelt's WPA Project. The WPA (Works Progress Administration) was designed to put people back to work during the Depression. The bandmaster's job was to set up a neighborhood kiddies' band to march in parades, especially the Portland Rose Festival parade. And that is how Burt Turner came to the Avenue.

Turner was a Johnny Appleseed in sweater vests, a stocky chain-smoking Music Man with a flair for John Philip Sousa, parades, and building a young person's self-esteem. He made being part of a marching band as important as being part of Little League, except nobody got cut and the parents, some of whom came to rehearsals, never lost their cool. "Wearing that beanie was a badge of honor for the children of Williams," says Florence M. Mills, a trombone player in Burt Turner's band along with Sid Porter and Floyd Standifer. That was more than sixty years ago. "Even small children who were not even in the band came to rehearsal to watch and imitate. Burt would march up and down the street and it was quite a spectacle. The police would block the main street with cars. Burt was like a basketball coach who let everyone

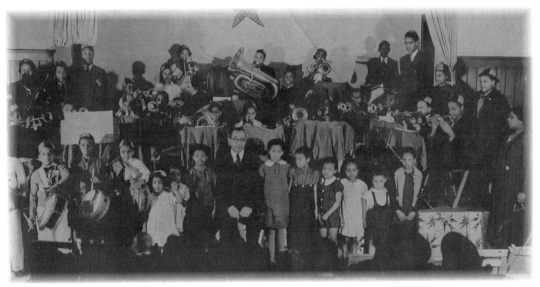

Burt Turner's WPA band

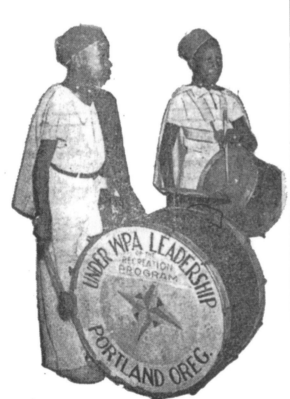

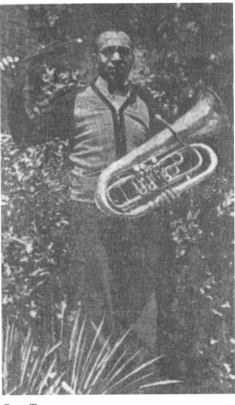

Burt Turner

(All photographs on this page courtesy of Florence Mills)

play regardless of their skill level. This fairness gave all the kids a chance to get better, and you know, none of those kids ever had a problem with the law or with drugs."[16]

With a variety of tricks and gimmicks, Burt Turner made a game out of learning scales and runs. "One of his big tricks was to give you an assignment like scales and you had to do it in front of everybody," says Standifer. "He played all the instruments—reeds, brass. He was an excellent teacher. His wife taught piano. Mr. Turner taught us in the basement of the YWCA on the corner of Tillamook and Williams and we played in the Portland Rose Festival parade each year with our little caps and stuff. When the movie *Alexander's Ragtime Band* came out, with Tyrone Power, they had our little band come to the Paramount Theater and we actually played 'Alexander's Ragtime Band' in front of everybody. They put me up on this box but the trumpet was so heavy they had to put a leather wrist band on to strengthen up my wrist so I could hold it. And that's how I got into it. Turner didn't seem to be a jazz player. I would from time to time just take off and alter the music a little bit because I was hearing other harmonies. All he would do was look at me like 'where did you get that?' But he never told me not to do it."[17]

Eighty or maybe ninety percent of the jazz music played at the Dude Ranch was based on the twelve-bar blues. Not the down-in-the-dumps country kind played on an acoustic guitar or harmonica but urban blues with horns, electric guitars, and more sophisticated lyrics. It was

played in three styles that often overlapped: bop, which had just arrived in Portland via Carl Thomas and a couple of piano players named Amadee and Brooks; boogie-woogie as played by Meade Lux Lewis; and jump.

Boogie-woogie was much more popular at the Dude Ranch than bop. Bop came out of New York and unless you were Bojangles, was not recommended for dancing. Boogie-woogie, on the other hand, was a byproduct of lumber camps and railroad yards. The repeated eight to the bar figures in the pianist's left hand echo a train rumbling over tracks.[18] Boogie-woogie was workingman's music, music that could substitute for a whole band when things got tough. It was down to earth, as is the history of the word itself. To boogie today is to dance in a lively manner. A century ago, in certain parts of the South, boogie-woogie meant syphilis and later sexual intercourse.[19]

Meade Lux Lewis revived the style in 1938 with his huge hit, "Honky Tonk Train." The popularity of boogie-woogie went beyond the piano. For a while every orchestra, no matter the size or style, had to have a boogie-woogie arrangement. But it was the jump bands that got the most out of the boogie-woogie eight to the bar feel, jump bands like Louis Jordan's Tympany Five, which came into being about the same time as boogie-woogie's revival.[20]

Jump evolved from big bands such as those of Lucky Millinder and particularly Lionel Hampton, whose early 1940s bands were incubators for jump leaders like Jack McVea, Earl Bostic, Arnett Cobb, and Louis Jordan himself. Like the big bands they came from, these little bands used repeated phrases called riffs when they were backing up soloists. Jump tries to do with three horns and a rhythm section what a sixteen-piece band does—and for a lot less money, making them very popular with agents and ballroom managers during the shortages and rations of World War II. They began to phase out in the mid-fifties. Tab Smith, Earl Bostic, and Johnny Otis were among the final acts. All of them played on the Avenue. Locally the very popular Hamiltones were an extension of the jump era.

The jitterbugs were the jump groups' reason for being. "Everything that got in the way of that," says swing expert Stanley Dance, "was pared away."[21] Veteran saxophonist Art Chaney once said if he couldn't get the dancers out on the floor, he took it personally. "We were insulted and don't think we didn't let them know it."[22]

Great bands inspire great dancers and visa versa. The best dancer on the Avenue was Tate Bay, a wall-eyed, five-by-five man with a club foot. Originally from Gary, Indiana, he landed here in 1945 and quickly became a favorite at the Dude Ranch and at McElroy's, an independently owned ballroom downtown at SW 4th and Main. The veteran jazz broadcaster Ray Horn was also a competitive swing dancer in those days and remembers Tate vividly.

He was the best I ever saw around these parts. I mean guys would come from Boise and Seattle to take him on but he was too slick.

He had what they called the New York style. No one could keep up with his casual but quicker than lightning moves. He'd do a running floor slide, overhead snatches, and his competition would end up like everyone else, standing in a circle watching. When he and his partner got too heated up, the crowd would cool them off by getting out their handkerchiefs and waving them.

He danced like he had some of that Empire Green that porters used to bring in. Women used to line up waiting for him to arrive and, get this, he was short and odd looking; one leg was six inches longer than the other, but it didn't seem to matter because he could always make everyone around him feel so good with that howling laugh of his and that cigar hanging out of his mouth. He could think up things to say that would make you feel like a million dollars. One night right after I had just finished a jazz show, he walked up to me and said, 'Ray, you shouldn't be a DJ. You should be a preacher or a famous politician.'[23]

When his competitive dancing days were over, you could find Tate holding court at the Stadium McDonald's on West Burnside or practicing some new steps on the broken-down porch of his home, a dilapidated flat that used to sit fifty yards away from the center field fence of the Civic Stadium, now PGE Park, in direct line with home plate.

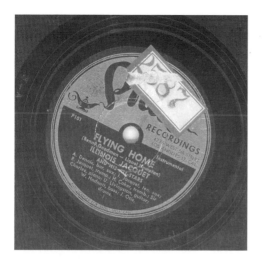
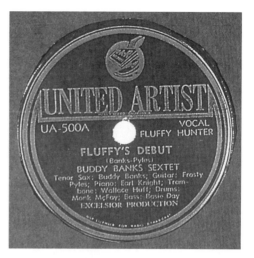

The tenor saxophone is king in the world of jump and what someone said about the trumpet in certain parts of New Orleans could also be said about the tenor saxophone at the Dude Ranch: "It practically blew itself." There was more talent in town on that instrument than on any other: Ralph Rosenlund, Don Brassfield, Roy Jackson, and later Kenny Hing, who played with Count Basie for many years. The main man at the Dude never even played there. Illinois Jacquet was from Texas and played the saxophone as if he'd heard Lester Young, Herschel Evans, and a few hellfire and damnation sermons. Lionel Hampton hired him in 1940 and let him loose on the 78 rpm Decca record called "Flyin' Home." The music world hasn't been the same since. In person he would get up from his chair, point the bell of his horn at the mike, and turn the place into a revival meeting, a mass orgy, the band riffing in the background like a congregation saying amen. People actually fainted. Some jazz writers now say that Illinois Jacquet's solos were the beginning of rock and roll. Perhaps, but it

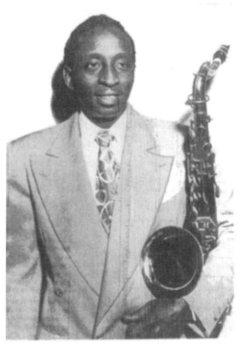

Buddy Banks (courtesy of McClendon family)

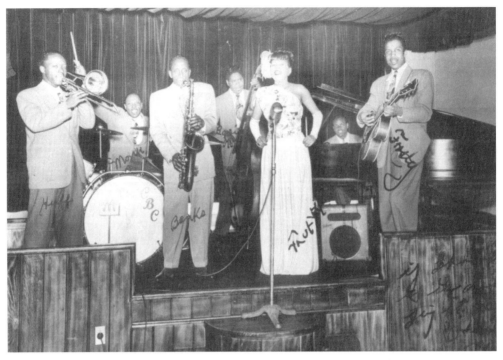

Buddy Banks band (courtesy of Bernice Slaughter)

sure did a lot for jump. Almost every tenor player at the Dude after that sounded a little like Illinois Jacquet. A few lucky jazz buffs got to hear Jacquet and Hampton at the Norse Hall. The Hall still stands at 111 NE 11th, the spacious ballroom and stage still in perfect condition, just the way it looked some sixty years ago when Lionel Hampton brought his Flyin' Home band into town with a veritable farm club of future jump stars.[24]

One of the best of the Jacquet-inspired jump bands was Buddy Banks and his Block Rhythms. It's hard to think of a group more popular at the Dude Ranch than Banks'. When he wasn't on Central Avenue in Los Angeles playing "Fluffy's Debut" and "Banks Boogie," he was at the Dude, sometimes for weeks in a row. There would always be a line waiting to

get in. His secret? A shrewd amalgamation of bop, boogie-woogie, and sassy vocals from Fluffy Hunter. The addition of a trombone made his group sound different from the rest, and Frosty Pyles, his guitar player, was a mix of Charlie Christian and T-Bone Walker.[25]

It's the bass player and the piano player, however, who are of the most interest to students of Portland jazz history. Basie Day, a gap-toothed happy-go-lucky owner of one of the great names in jazz (right up there with pianist Preston Keyes), stayed in Portland for the rest of his life. Not until the arrival of Leroy Vinnegar had there been a more in-demand bass player than Basie Day. Earl Knight, Buddy Banks's popular all-purpose piano player and organist, could also double on the tenor saxophone. One local reviewer compared this Floridian's

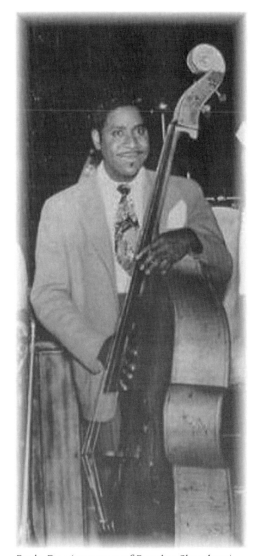

Basie Day (courtesy of Bernice Slaughter)

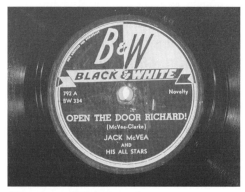

(Courtesy of Dick Cogan)

marvelous technique to Art Tatum,[26] but his albums in the 1950s with Jimmy Hamilton, Coleman Hawkins, and Lester Young reveal someone closer to Nat Cole. He played in Portland off and on for four or five years before moving to New York in hopes of studying at Juilliard.

Another Texas tenor was Jack McVea, who was very close to Illinois Jacquet, literally, since he sat next to him in the Hampton band during the recording of "Flyin' Home." Jack McVea also made his reputation with Norman Granz in Jazz at the Philharmonic with his solo on "Lester Leaps In." His act at the Dude was more entertainment than art, full of costumes and comedy routines. While he was playing at the Dude and the Vancouver Barracks, he wrote or actually compiled his biggest hit and one of the best-selling records of the decade, "Open the Door Richard!"[27] The title became a national catchphrase and the song was recorded many times—over fifteen versions in all.

The house band at the Dude for many weeks was the Banjoski Adams band, a jump group out of Seattle. It featured yet another Jacquet exponent named Tootie Boyd, who had played in Portland in the 1930s. As in the Buddy Banks band, two of Banjoski's sidemen became permanent members of the Portland jazz scene: one was Art Bradford, a short baby-faced show drummer with exceptional time and a deadpan stare. When he played musicals he never missed a cue. He was perfect for jump bands like Banjoski Adams' and later with the Hamiltones. "We were a group thing rather than any one individual," says Bradford. "We left rock and roll out of it completely because

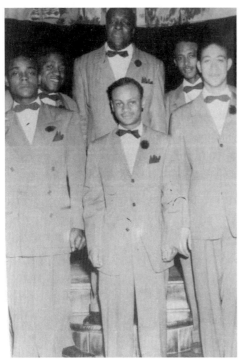

Banjoski Adams band at the Dude Ranch. Front row, left to right: Tootie Boyd, Art Bradford, Earl "Longoody" Austin. Leader Banjoski Adams is towering over Bradford in back. The two others on each side of him are unknown. (Courtesy of Bernice Slaughter)

if you don't feel it, best not to mess with it."[28] In the 1960s he would occasionally grace the rhythm section of Chris Tyle's superb swing band, Wholly Cats.

The other member of the Banjoski Adams band to make Portland his home was Earl "Longoody" Austin. He was not the showman that Basie Day was, but if you wanted a bass player who was easy to get along with and very dependable, knew all the chord changes, and could swing, then Longoody was the guy you wanted.

Before Longoody and Basie Day came to town, Portland was short on bass players. Hank Wales was the main bass player in Portland for years. Bonnie Addleman Wetzel and Keith Hodgson were living in Vancouver, Washington. Al Johnson along with Eddie Wied's brother Al were playing on the Avenue. There was no one even close to the artistry of Red Callender, who had recorded with Lester Young, Nat Cole, Louis Armstrong, and Norman Granz's Jazz at the Philharmonic, before arriving in Portland with his trio to play at the Dude Ranch and the Vancouver Barracks.

McClendon, writing in his *Observer*, told all the bass players in town to be sure to hear this phenomenon. Hank Wales thought they had seen it all when Jimmy Blanton visited the Clover Club in 1941 after his performance with Duke Ellington at the Civic Auditorium. But Callender, also a composer and a tuba player, went beyond that. Far enough to be Charlie Mingus's first teacher, and before Red Mitchell and Leroy Vinnegar, the most dominant bass player on the West Coast. He ended up being on almost as many recordings as the prolific Leroy Vinnegar.[29]

Equally appealing to the sporting crowd at the Dude Ranch was Callender's pianist, Duke Brooks. Brooks was an early admirer of Bud Powell and one of the first bop piano players to visit Portland.[30] His assignment with the Callender band was to play a little like Nat King Cole, whose trio recordings the Callender group was emulating in arrangements like "Honeysuckle Rose" and Cecil Gant's "I Wonder." Duke Brooks can be heard to greater advantage two years later on some of

Teddy Edwards's first saxophone recordings. Edwards, a bop pioneer, says, "I can't think of a warmer player. He was killed hoboing his way to St. Louis to see his mother. He was the kind of person who could stay away from home only so long." [31]

It was only fitting that the Dude opened its doors on May 29, 1945 to the sounds of Al Pierre and his orchestra. Pierre was truly one of the pioneers of Portland jazz, belonging in the same room with Don Anderson, Monte Ballou, and a few others. In the 1930s, Pierre was everywhere, as the slogan goes, from the posh and polished ballrooms of

Portland's finest golf clubs to the funky quarters of Albina Hall on Russell. Pierre was the Tom Grant of his time and the first person society matrons, prom planners, and nightclub owners thought of when they wanted a well-dressed, well-rehearsed band, one that played sweet and hot. Don't think that Pierre didn't have some pretty serious competition: there were Billy Webb and His Syncopaters, Louis Richardson and the Playmates. The Melody Boys were playing at Henry Thiele's and Burt Turner and his wife had the Dixieland Strollers, but Pierre had the best musicians in town because he paid them more.

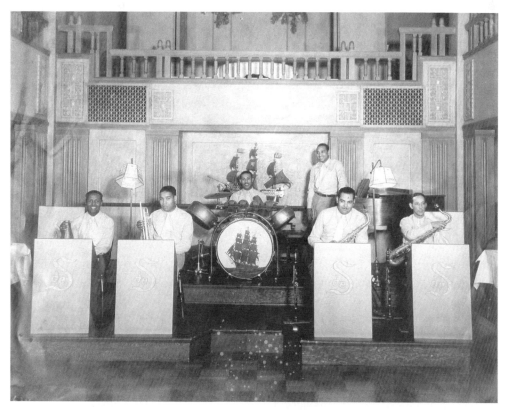

Al Pierre band. Left to right: Russ Jones, Jimmy Adams, Charles Wilson, Al Pierre (standing). Last two sax players are unknown. (Courtesy of Arthur Prentice Studio and Cleve Williams)

At the Dude, Pierre featured Seattle's Jabbo Ward on tenor saxophone and the influential drummer Vern Brown, who advertised himself as "the best time around." Al Pierre taught some of his sidemen to read music. One was Portland's "Prince of the Blues," Clarence Williams. "He was such a class act and an excellent piano player. Not modern, but very, very good. He was the leader of us all. He taught me how to be a working musician, how to be professional, being on time and properly dressed. Something your normal music teacher never gets around to telling you. His mother was an accomplished musician of her own. She taught Al to read by just using the fingers of his right hand; a baby could learn to do it. I couldn't even read whole notes before I met Al. He showed me the five finger approach to reading music and it changed my whole approach to playing the blues. Ask anyone alive about Al Pierre. They'll tell you," Williams recalls.[32]

Al Pierre originally came from Tacoma, where his grandparents had moved to escape laws of slavery. He worked in California for a while in the 1920s before coming to Portland. He opened the Frat Hall in 1930 with a violin in his band. In 1932 his growing number of fans could find Al and his orchestra propped up against the wall of a speakeasy on the fourth floor of a downtown building owned by racketeer Swede Ferguson.[33] In 1934 he and his band were regulars at Blue Lake Park under the name Harlem Blue Knights. And all the while he was holding down one of the best and longest weekend engagements—twelve years at Berg's Chalet, located by the King Tower in Southwest Portland. Eventually Pierre went to Alaska in the 1950's and then back to Seattle, where he had lived during the 1940s. He finally died there of hardening of the arteries, an affliction, historian Tom Stoddard says, caused by "too many wild women and too many thick steaks."[34]

Except for the Hamiltones, jump pretty much disappeared from Portland by the mid-fifties. It was taken over by doo-wop vocal groups, grandstanding guitarists, and exhibitionist tenor saxophonists as the music turned from rhythm and blues to rock and roll. In the late nineties, jump enjoyed a brief revival. Its home in Portland was the newly renovated Crystal Ballroom on West Burnside.[35] As for the Dude Ranch, it was closed down in 1946. The papers said it was all that big time gambling and an accidental shooting. Most people think it was the mixed couples, the flirting, those racy dances, those happy bottoms "shakin' the African."

CHAPTER 2

The Castle Jazz Band

Jon Hendricks, the poet laureate of jazz, might say that the Dude Ranch was so nice that it had to be opened twice. Sam Amato and a partner opened the Dude Ranch for the first time in May of 1944. The increasing demand for Black talent in what was becoming a predominantly Black neighborhood was one of the reasons that Amato sold the Dude Ranch to Charles Patterson in the middle of May 1945. Most of the music in the first edition was by Herman Jobelmann, a symphonic bassist who led an easy-listening group playing rumbas, foxtrots, and waltzes.[1] The jazz that was played at the Dude Ranch in its first incarnation was by Monte Ballou. Stop anyone on the corner of SW Broadway and Salmon in the forties and fifties. Ask them who it is that best personifies jazz in Portland, and nine out of ten would tell you Monte Ballou and his Castle Jazz Band, named after the Castle near Oregon City.[2]

The Castle is still standing, albeit in serious disrepair, about a block west of TeBo's Restaurant, where McLoughlin and River Road come together. In the thirties it was a roadhouse tavern made out of hand-cut stone by an imported French stonecutter, complete with turrets, arched windows, medieval doors, and a tower, which was removed later.[3]

The Castle Jazz Band was an all-white group of excellent musicians playing music by Black musicians of the teens and twenties. It was and still is the most popular jazz group ever to come out of Portland, with fan clubs as far away as The Netherlands and Argentina.

They were part of a worldwide New Orleans revival. Portland and especially San Francisco were citadels. Most people called it Dixieland, but San Franciscan band leaders Bob Scobey, Lu Watters, and Turk Murphy thought of themselves as neotraditionalists. They were fed up with the state of jazz in the forties. Some people didn't like the over-arranged riffs of swing bands even when Louis Armstrong was leading them.[4] A few weren't too sure of Eddie Condon and his Chicago-style jazz. Beboppers were drug-addicted crackpots who ought to be wiped off the face of jazz. The proponents of this revival wanted to return to the roots of jazz, to the rules and standards and instrumentations of its originators: Jelly Roll Morton, Buddy Bolden, Freddie Keppard, King Oliver, and Sidney Bechet. There were no saxophones, no guitars, no string bass in the Castle Jazz Band; instead, a trumpet, clarinet, trombone in the front line and a rhythm section of a tuba, drums, banjo, and piano. Many expert musicians

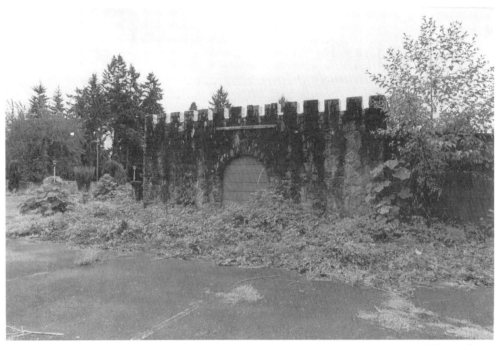

The Castle in 2005 (courtesy of the author)

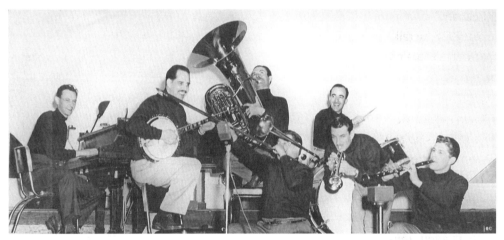

Monte Ballou and the Castle Jazz Band. Left to right: Larry DuFresne, Monte Ballou, Bob Short, George Bruns, Homer Welch, Don Kinch, Bob Gilbert (courtesy of Ted Hallock)

traveled through the Castle Jazz Band in its many editions: drummers Axel Tyle and Homer Welch; Bob Short, the tuba player; and clarinetists Bob Gilbert and Willy Pavia.

The most successful member of the Castle Jazz Band was trombone player George Bruns, a six-foot-four, big-boned country boy from Sandy, Oregon. Bruns's stoic countenance and sleepy-eyed stare belied his extraordinary talents. He left Ballou and the gang in 1950 and went to California to play with Turk Murphy, but ended up in Hollywood as Walt Disney's music man, turning out over two hundred animated pictures while composing award-winning songs, including one of the best-selling hits in popular music, "The Ballad of Davy Crockett."

In 1978 he talked about this experience in a newspaper article.

In 1955 I was doing a TV show for Walt Disney, which was Davy Crockett, so Walt comes up to me one day and says, "George, instead of those time lapses between the episodes why don't you write a little throwaway song with a little verse." I went home and wrote this little ditty in about thirty minutes, but when the show's director heard it the next day, he said to me, "That's no good. Get rid of it." But the next morning Walt comes up to me again and he asks me to sing it and I did. So Walt says, "See, George? I can't tell much by your singing but I think we might have something here." I arranged it for the orchestra and Walt went absolutely crazy over it. When that thing hit the charts it was like a dam breaking.

They went nuts over it in New York, everywhere. It was on the hit parade for twenty-eight straight weeks. It ended up selling over eight million copies. But still, you know, I loved playing with that Castle Jazz Band. We never paid ourselves. We left the money in the kitty. But we got better and better, and at the Ratskeller on SW Taylor and Broadway when Monte would go into "The Old Green River," the place would go crazy.[5]

The high point of the Castle Jazz Band was the 1949 Dixieland Jubilee in Los Angeles put on by impresario Gene Norman. It was billed as the world series of jazz, and the biggest names in the traditional jazz field were there: Firehouse Five, Kid Ory, Bob Crosby's Bobcats, Bud Freeman, Muggsy Spanier—but it was Portland's own Castle Jazz Band that won the hearts of the crowd with its rendition of "High Society." "People liked us better than the Bobcats or even Kid Ory. We were really tops then," says cornetist Don Kinch, one of the big reasons for the success of the Castle Jazz Band.

I got into the Castle Jazz Band right after the war but it was going on way back in the thirties when Axel Tyle was there; what a great drummer he was. And Willy Pavia at the Castle on River Road. Anyway we made some of our first recordings in a cabinet shop with homemade recording gear, and one of them on the Castle label was called "Floating Down the Old Green River." It caught on nationally with sales in the millions, and because of that Monte bought the Diamond Horseshoe which was on top of the Liberty Theater

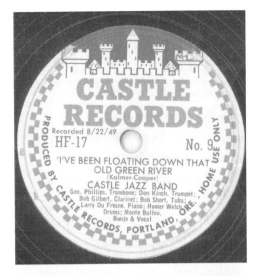

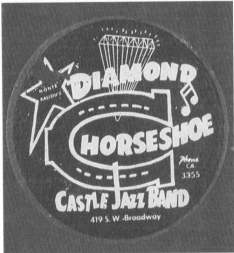

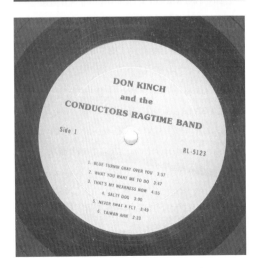

there on Broadway. Of course, the Bank of California is sitting there today.

Don't get Kinch started on bebop. "I can't stand bebop and Louis Armstrong couldn't either or Tommy Dorsey. To me its very unmusical. What are they trying to say? It's beyond me." And Kinch doesn't like the word "jazz" either.

Anything that isn't symphony or country or cowboy is jazz, according to some of these so-called jazz radio stations. I hate the word "Dixieland" too. It conjures up old men with straw hats playing rickity-tickity and all that jazzamatazz highnoting horseshit stuff. New Orleans music is different. It's your sound that matters, and how your sound blends in with other sounds, and how it weaves in and out. That's everything to me. Guys like Willy Pavia, God he could create a beautiful sound. And that's what it is all about, the blending of sounds, the ensemble. The sound of Louis Armstrong and King Oliver. That's jazz.[6]

Kinch left town for a while to make some records with the famous Turk Murphy band in San Francisco, most notably *Barrelhouse Jazz*, an early Columbia LP. In the late 1970s, he formed a ragtime band called the Conductors that was very popular in Old Town. Kinch took that group into a studio in the late 1970s and made an LP. One of the tracks was a tribute to Freddie Keppard called "Salty Dog."

CHAPTER 3

Struttin' at the Golden West

Freddie Keppard was a high-note trumpeter with a hot temper. He was called King Keppard because he was, after Buddy Bolden, the second trumpet king of New Orleans, which was a little like being footballer Jim Brown in Cleveland in 1964. Keppard was tall with broad shoulders, a swaggering walk, and the diaphragm of a long-distance swimmer. He was handsome and reckless, and many women where he worked made themselves available. Long before Louis Armstrong, he was among the first to use a handkerchief when he played, pretending to hide his secret technique from his competitors. He was also one of the first to popularize the Harmon mute, later identified with Miles Davis.[1]

Portland heard jazz for the first time, before it was even called jazz, when Keppard and the Original Creole Orchestra took the stage at the Pantages Theater on the corner of SW Alder and Broadway. It happened sometime after 1:00 a.m. Monday, November 23, 1914.[2] As a vaudeville act, the OCO were the original Jazz Messengers. They were the first group to spread this new way of playing music across the United States. Art Pantages hired them himself after hearing Keppard's powerhouse cornet during an intermission at a boxing match

in Los Angeles. The OCO played fifteen-minute performances each day as part of a show, backing up semi-classical singers, Black-faced minstrels, and comedians, and presumably playing a little jazz, crude as it would sound to our ears, "like the musical counterpart of man's first attempt at flight," said an eminent jazz historian.[3]

The tour took them all the way to New York, where around 1916 RCA Victor asked them to make the first jazz record. Keppard said, "no," for a number of reasons that boiled down to vanity.[4] He apparently wanted to be paid as much as RCA Victor leading star, Enrico Caruso. That decision would compromise Keppard's place in jazz history, that and his leaving New Orleans too early to be an influence on jazz's greatest soloist, Louis Armstrong.

Freddie Keppard did not make a record until ten years after he was in Portland. According to his biggest fans, Jelly Roll Morton and Mutt Carey, he was way past his prime. He didn't sound anything like the way he played when he was with the Original Creole Orchestra. By 1924 he'd become a desperate alcoholic playing in an outworn style.[5] Armstrong's innovations had left him in the dust. Because of this, less is known of Keppard than of Buddy Bolden, King

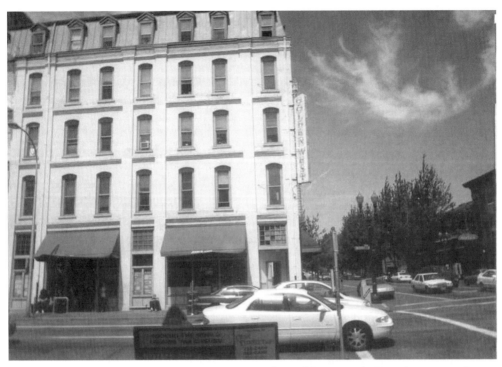

The Golden West in 2005 (courtesy of Ron Weber)

Oliver, or any other early New Orleans trumpet kings. There are no books on Freddie Keppard. Frequently he is omitted from jazz history courses. Sometimes he is absent in general overviews of the history of the trumpet in jazz. What is known of Freddie Keppard would have you believe that this Creole trumpeter was larger than life. His tone was supposed to be more beautiful than Harry James's. His cornet was so powerful that he could shake walls. One writer claims that while drunk one night in the middle of winter, he fell asleep, freezing the entire left side of his face. Worse, the next morning he fell down a flight of stairs and bloodied his lips, yet he brought down the house that very evening with a barrage of high notes unheard of until then.[6]

Freddie and the orchestra stayed at the Golden West Hotel on the corner of NW Everett and Broadway. It stands there today as a low-cost hotel. In 1914 it was the center of Black social events, where all Black entertainers stayed. But more than that, in the words of the owner W. D. Allen, "a hotel convenient for railroad and shipyard workers of such quality that New York can not boast of such a fine Black hotel."[7] The Golden West had Turkish baths, a gymnasium, a fine restaurant, a candy shop, and in the basement, pool tables and a barber shop owned by Waldo Bogle (former city commissioner Dick Bogle's grandfather). There was a gambling room and bar where there was always live music and where the Original Creole Orchestra with Freddie Keppard would always have a

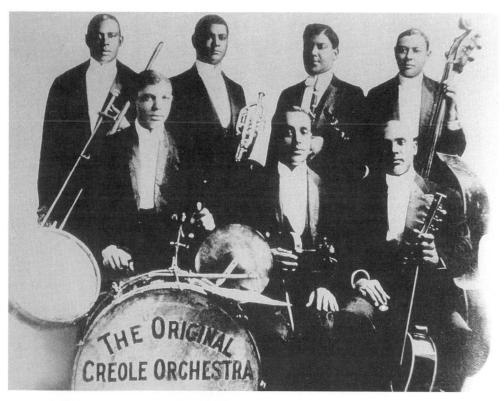

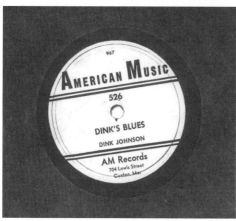

Left to right, front row: Dink Johnson, James Palao, Leon Williams; back row: Eddie Venson, Freddie Keppard, George Baquet, Bill Johnson (courtesy of Hogan archives)

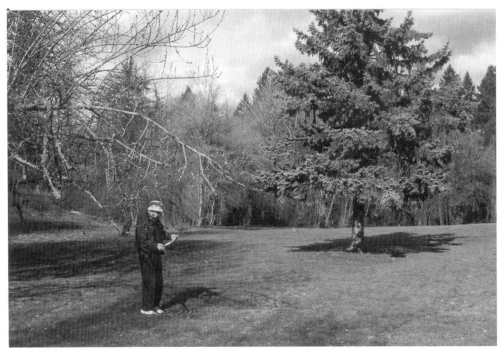

*Author looking for Dink Johnson's grave
(courtesy of Bob Trowbridge)*

chance to tear loose without the constraints of their vaudeville responsibilities.

Freddie Keppard was not the whole show. Leon Williams and James Palao, the guitar player and violinist, were worthy constituents. Eddie Venson was a popular tailgate trombone player. Clarinetist George Baquet recorded with Jelly Roll Morton. Bill Johnson was one of the first in jazz to play pizzicato bass. His brother Dink Johnson was not only one of the first drummers in jazz, but more importantly a future resident of Portland.

Though Portland has done little to remember him, Jelly Roll Morton's brother-in-law, Dink Johnson, is the city's most valuable jazz figure. He was among the first to take the New Orleans style of drumming on the road with the Original Creole Orchestra.[8] In 1945 he made a

series of records on the American label that drew attention among fans of barrelhouse piano. In 1950 he moved to Portland, and in 1954, as a reward for all his achievements, he was dumped in an unmarked grave in an abandoned cemetery. It takes a guide and a road map to find him.

Besides drums and piano, Dink Johnson was the clarinetist on one of the most historically significant records in jazz history. The Kid Ory Sunshine Band recordings of 1922 were the first by a Black jazz group and the first jazz recordings made on the West Coast, setting a style that would eventually reach Portland. More than that, these recordings were the first accurate examples of New Orleans jazz played by the pioneers themselves. One critic called it the beginning of an American art form

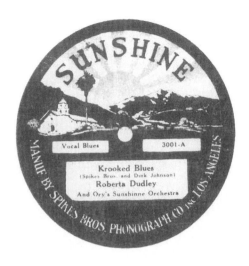

It was Dink Johnson's brother-in-law, the legendary Jelly Roll Morton, who convinced Dink to give up the clarinet and become a full-time piano player. Telling them apart on a record can be difficult.[10]

And Dink could cook, literally. He had a restaurant in California for a while that was famous for its rice and beans, a dish he learned from his sister, Anita, Jelly Roll's main love in life. A severe arthritis and stomach problem prevented Dink from playing much piano in Portland. So instead he became the Creole cook at Monte Ballou's Diamond Horseshoe Restaurant. You have to wonder what was going through Dink's mind when the Castle Jazz Band would open each night with "Ory's Creole Trombone," one of the selections Dink played on the original 1922 Sunshine label.[11]

As Dink's health declined, he began drinking more and more while hanging out at a bar not far from his brother's house on SE Hawthorne. Dink, like Jelly Roll, was a big talker, especially after a few beers. So one night he was waxing on to the bartender about his piano prowess, about the good old days with Freddie Keppard, and all about Jelly Roll's first trip to Portland in 1920. A party at a table close by seemed fascinated. "If they could find a piano, could he play a little for them?" one of them asked. "Find that piano and let the good times roll," Dink was reported to have said. It was a setup. Once they were in the car and on their way, they beat him up, stole seventeen dollars out of his wallet, tore off his pants, and left his half nude body lying in a heap on North Larrabee Street. He

like James Whistler's painting, *The White Girl*, or some of James Fenimore Cooper's descriptions of the American landscape.[9] The value of these recordings as an American original did not escape Hal Smith, a drummer and former Portlander. In the 1980s he ran a Dixieland group called Hal Smith and the Creole Sunshine Band. On the back of their first album, there is a photocopy of the original Sunshine label showing the title, "Krooked Blues" by Dink Johnson.

Before Dink moved to Portland in 1950, the invaluable jazz writer Floyd Levin interviewed him about those famous recordings. "I was actually a drummer, you know," says Dink, "I always wanted to play clarinet since hearing Larry Shields with the Original Dixieland Jazz Band. So I borrowed a horn from the Spike Brothers' store, and I practiced every day, trying to sound like Shields. Kid Ory's regular player for some reason couldn't make the gig in Santa Monica, so Ory asked me to substitute. You know," Dink added, "I don't remember if I ever returned the clarinet."

never recovered, and the following November he died.[12]

In a book called *Jazz on Record, a Critical Guide to Jazz Recordings*, Peter Gammond, a British writer, said this: "Dink Johnson is one of the rare vintages of jazz, a special liquor to be brought out after the coffee and brandy of other traditional jazz pianists. He was no great shakes technically, but his recordings are so uniquely enjoyable and delightful, that it is hard to imagine anyone who likes jazz not getting a great kick out of them."

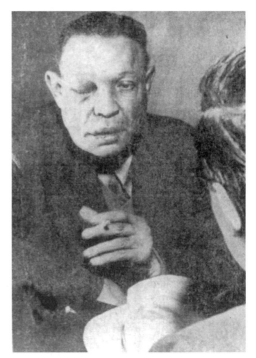

Dink Johnson after the attack that took his life (courtesy of Oregon Journal, *1954)*

CHAPTER 4

The Acme: Rebop Spoken There

When the Black and Tan Dude Ranch closed in the fall of 1946, another club called the Dude Ranch opened up on Union Avenue. It had little in common with its predecessor except that it was also a target for city officials, who eventually closed it.[1] After that, the place to be was on the second floor of a two-story wooden building on the corner of North Cherry Court, just about where the Ramada Inn sits today. In the thirties it was called the Ballot Box. Owner Charlie Garrett, founder of Madrona Records, was the shrewdest Black businessman in Portland next to Tom Johnson. The upstairs had heavy gambling and Sunday jam sessions. The bar downstairs looked like one of those wild west saloons you see in cowboy movies of the thirties, complete with brass railing, a spittoon, a gentleman's relief trough, a billy club under the cash register, and one of those oversized mirrors on the back wall behind the bar. That was so Charlie Garrett could check out the "pretty foxes" coming and going. From the back seat of his car one night, one of them, in a fit of jealousy, put a bullet through his head and got away with it.[2]

That was a couple of years after a fraternal organization bought the Ballot Box in 1943, modernizing the bar and painting the walls and ceilings. They dressed the waitresses and barmaids in short black skirts and called it the Acme Club. Jazz people called it the House of Rebop because the earliest stirrings of this music was first heard there.[3]

The first Portland musician to play in this new idiom, soon to be forever called bebop, was North Fargo Street's Carl Thomas. Every large city on the West Coast had its version of Charlie Parker, who was to modern jazz what Bunk Johnson was to the neotraditionalists. San Francisco had Pony Poindexter; Los Angeles had Sonny Criss; Seattle had Roscoe Weathers. Portland had Carl Thomas. He played in Portland for ten years off and on before joining rhythm and blues star Lloyd Price.[4] He returned in 1970, sitting in on tenor saxophone with Billy Larkin and Warren Bracken, and at Sidney's with the dynamic Mary Field. Thomas died in obscurity in Seattle without ever being recognized as the pioneer of Portland bebop. Alto saxophonist Les Williams and other members of the Thomas legacy insist that Thomas was playing something close to bop by the end of 1944. This was even before the first Charlie Parker and Dizzy Gillespie records came out. One theory was that he discovered it while he was playing in a restaurant in Oakland that was owned by his mother. Another was

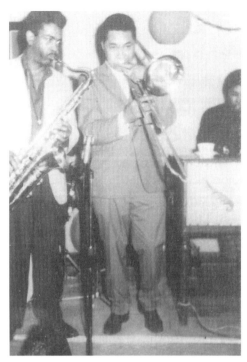

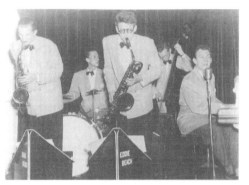

Ed Beach quintet (courtesy of Lee Rockey)

The return of Carl Thomas (left) with Cleve Williams (courtesy of Cleve Williams)

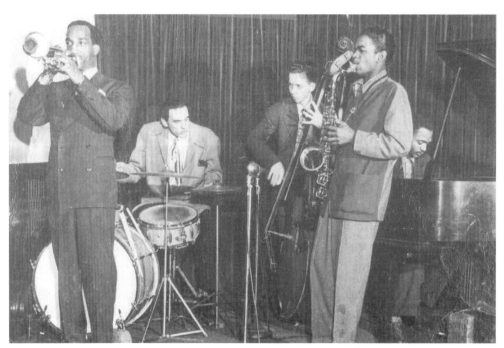

Left to right: Skeeter Evans, J. Parker, Keith Hodgson, Carl Thomas, "Brownie" Amadee (courtesy of Lee Rockey)

that he had been in the audience at McElroy's when Sonny Stitt came through with Tiny Bradshaw.[5]

In any case, Thomas was the first in the city to play in this new style where the lines were longer, the harmonies more advanced, and the beat had shifted from the bass drum to something called the ride cymbal. In bop all the accents seemed to be in the wrong place. It stopped and started at breakneck speeds and the musicians had to know all the right chord changes to the most frequently played popular songs. Dexter Gordon, the Hall of Fame tenor saxophonist, once said, "Bebop is the music of the future."[6] John Hammond called it "a collection of nauseating clichés." Louis Armstrong hated it; so did George Frazier, the *Down Beat* critic. Sportswriter Jimmy Cannon said, "The sound of bop is like being inside a china shop in an earthquake."[7] Magazines caricatured it or patronized it; *Life* ran an article on the goatees, the berets, the handshake, and other manifestations of the bop cult. One of the few critics to publicly support bebop in the beginning was Leonard Feather.[8]

Before Ed Beach was a famous disc jockey, "creating a generation of people who are now keeping jazz alive," he played piano and led a group of some of the most talented young white musicians in Portland: Marty Wright, Lee Rockey, and one of the future stars of West Coast jazz, Bill Hood. "Christ, it was 1946 and what did we know about bop," says Beach. "Those first Gillespie and Parker sides playing 'Hothouse' and 'Groovin' High' had just come out, and we were

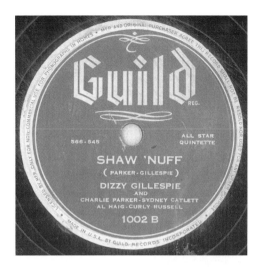

trying to memorize every nuance on those records. But nobody was really playing it. And Jesus, one night this Black cat comes in and we stood still. My God, we had never heard anything like that in person." It was Carl Thomas.[9]

Carl's favorite piano player at the Acme was a quiet round-faced fellow called Leo "Dark Eyes" Amadee. He came to Portland in late 1943 as an army private from New Orleans by way of San Bernadino. When he arrived, he was a boogie-woogie specialist. After hearing Monk at the Dude, he began to absorb the elements of modern piano and evolved a way of playing that resembled the sparse style of John Lewis on the early Charlie Parker Savoy records.[10] He left for San Francisco in 1948 to become a house pianist at Jimbo's Bop City, but not before introducing many young aspiring pianists to the world of Monk and Bud Powell. His influence on jazz piano and particularly on Lorraine Walsh Geller cannot be underestimated. She would be Portland's proto-bopper.

Walsh was a tall red-haired bebopper in her senior year at Washington High

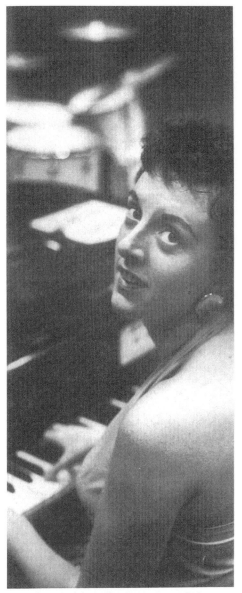

Lorraine Walsh Geller (courtesy of Claxton archives)

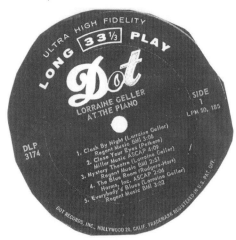

School when she would show up at the Acme or Jackie's Cafe, listening to the man whose chord progressions and subtle rhythms she worked hours to emulate. When she died of a pulmonary infection in 1958, she was only thirty. She had already played with Stan Getz, Dizzy Gillespie, Zoot Sims, Miles Davis, and Charlie Parker. Even in that league she was exceptional. Anybody who ever shared the stage with her would tell you that and make no concessions about gender.[11]

One of the easiest ways to hurt Walsh would be to tell her that she played well for a "girl." You heard that a lot in the forties and fifties, not only about her but about other exciting pianists like Marian McPartland, Barbara Carroll, and the venerable Mary Lou Williams. Sometimes the prejudice towards women instrumentalists reached ludicrous proportions. Band leader Earl Whitney, who hired her, likes to tell about the time his group lost a job because a nightclub owner didn't like her looks.

We'd got this call for an audition at the Tropics Club so we went out there and played. When it was over, the owner called me over to the bar and said, "You kids sound nice, but the girl doesn't look good on stage. She's gotta go." He never said anything about the way she played.

I didn't take the job of course, and I never told Lorraine about it. She was just one of the guys to us. In fact, we all called her "man." It must have gotten under her skin though, 'cause one day she called me over and said, "Look, Earl,

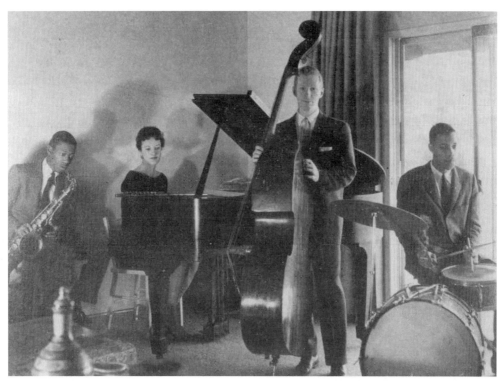

Lorraine Walsh Geller with the Red Mitchell Quartet, 1957: left to right, James Clay, Geller, Red Mitchell, Billy Higgins (courtesy of Ray Avery)

I'm no man, I'm a woman." From then on we called her "Jazz." Pretty soon everybody in town was calling her that.[12]

From 1948 to 1949, "Jazz" Walsh was everywhere. She didn't have a steady job. It would be the Freddie Keller Big Band at the old Uptown Ballroom one night and the Chicken Coop off Sandy Boulevard the next. She seemed obsessed, practicing and listening to records all day and jamming all night. No wonder they called her "Jazz."

Singer Jeannie Hackett, Walsh's best friend at Washington High School, recalls those wild times over a half a century ago. "I don't know how we survived. Sometimes we played for three days and

nights at a time. Lorraine would just keep going until the bass player's fingertips would start to bleed. We used to haunt all the record shops, too, looking for Nat King Cole and Gene Krupa records. I don't know why but Lorraine always liked Krupa's pianist, Teddy Napoleon. Ed and Mabel Walsh had Lorraine late in life. She was an only child, and they acted like they were amazed at what they had spawned."[13]

Nobody really knows how Walsh discovered jazz. Her old friend Jack Hasbrouck says that the first time he ever heard her play was at a Franklin High School assembly in 1942. "She was playing in a boogie-woogie quartet with George Cole, and then later on she accompanied the very popular singer Johnnie Ray, who went on to make all these hit records about crying in the early fifties. I used to take my Art Tatum and Teddy Wilson records over to her house on SE Ankeny. I couldn't believe how supportive her parents were, especially her mother, who used to pick up on all the hippest bop expressions. I remember one day she said to me: 'Hey Jack, we had a ball last night. Lorraine was really swinging.' I went into the service after that, and when I got out, I remember she had already heard Bud Powell and was well into bebop."[14]

She also had been studying with the piano patriarch of Portland, Gene Confer, who remembered her as the most anxious student he ever had. Confer remembered her getting so pumped up before her lessons that he thought she would actually pass out on the keyboard.

No one ever wanted to become a first-rate jazz musician more than Walsh did. She was willing to pay for it too. The perceptive composer, Ernie Hood, remembered her attention to details: "I heard Lorraine back in 1947. I noticed even then that Lorraine never took the cheap shortcuts other pianists did to make up for the strength it takes to play rapidly. She was very strong and never repeated herself like other pianists who are just getting started in the field. Lorraine was never satisfied, but I was thrilled, especially at the immense thinking that went into each chord. I knew then that she was going to be great."[15]

In 1949 she joined the Sweethearts of Rhythm, an integrated, all-woman road band that played one-night stands all over America. Six women in a station wagon, sometimes for five hundred miles at a stretch, is no easy way to make a buck. They survived on cheese and crackers and four hours of sleep. In most cities, they stayed in the Black districts, where Walsh learned how to play the blues. Her favorite tune in those days was Avery Parrish's "After Hours," which she learned to play with great sensitivity and timing.

Integrated bands were taboo in the South. To get around this, Walsh and the other white band members put on black makeup to make themselves look like mulattos. Most of the time it worked. However tenor saxophonist Willene Barton remembers once in Louisiana when it didn't: "This policeman looked in the stage door and said, 'Well, I don't know whether you're black or not, but I suggest that you guys get out of town fast.' We did too. It was hard, sometimes dangerous. We'd probably still be in jail today."[16]

Walsh left the Sweethearts in 1952 but not before she had met the love of her life, alto saxophonist Herb Geller. They were married in New York City in March of that year, and thus began one of the most successful husband-and-wife alliances in the history of jazz, right up there with Red Norvo and Mildred Bailey or Louis Armstrong and Lil Armstrong. Shortly after that, Herb Geller joined the Billy May band while Lorraine Geller gigged around New York with her friend, Bonnie Wetzel. When the Billy May band returned to its base in Los Angeles, the Gellers moved with them.

Los Angeles in the early fifties was a jazz players' paradise. There were nightclubs, lots of studio work and recording opportunities, but you had to have a union card, which required a six-month waiting period. Of course, you could always play the strip joints, and that's what the Gellers did to support themselves while Lorraine Geller was waiting for her card. The most infamous of these was Duffy's Gaiety, near Hollywood and Vine. Lenny Bruce was the main act; his wife Honey was the stripper. Lorraine and Herb Geller backed them up. In a taped interview from his home in Hamburg, Germany, Herb Geller talked about those days in Los Angeles:

Working at Duffy's was something else. All the top musicians and show people were there. I remember once the Miles Davis drummer Philly Joe Jones sat in with us. That's when Lenny taught him that Bela Lugosi routine that he used on his record called "Blues for Dracula." Bruce was at the height of his career. His material was fresh, his improvisations brilliant. He always felt there was a natural affinity between jazz and comedy. He used to try out his acts on us. If we laughed, it was great. He didn't care if the audience dug it or not as long as the musicians liked it. Lorraine had a great sense of humor and drama. That used to come out when she was backing up Lenny on the piano. He'd go into a monologue based on what he'd read in the newspaper that day, and Lorraine would play these mock fills in the background—real schmaltzy stuff based on "Humoresque" or some other well-known classical piece. It would just break Lenny up, right in the middle of his act. They inspired each other. He was really knocked out by her accompaniment; and of course, she and I loved his humor.[17]

The burlesque theaters put food on the Gellers' table, but Lorraine Geller craved a steady diet of jazz. She began sitting in at Zardi's on Monday nights, Terry Lester's Jazz Cellar on Wednesdays, and the famous Lighthouse at Hermosa Beach on Sundays, where she eventually became the house pianist. By consensus of the best and the brightest of the Los Angeles jazz circles, this "proto-bopper" from Portland was a hot prospect. Jazz writers compared her with Horace Silver, Bud Powell, and Joe Albany. Trumpeters Maynard Ferguson and Shorty Rogers asked her to record with them. So did the award-winning bassist Red Mitchell, who said about her at the time: "One of Lorraine's great qualities is her overall feeling, which goes beyond her playing. When she's backing a soloist, she's very good about getting a unanimous feeling, not playing so much so as to inhibit anybody, but just the right amount."[18]

The biggest musical thrill was the time she sat in with the co-inventor of modern jazz, Charlie "Yardbird" Parker. Bird had caught Geller at the Lighthouse, liked her style and asked her to play a couple of dance jobs with him at the 5/4 Ballroom in the Watts District of Los Angeles. But at the last minute, he hired another pianist who had been unemployed for over a year and desperately needed the job.

Herb Geller remembers when Parker called to apologize:

Bird called and said he was sorry about the whole thing, and Lorraine said don't worry about it, and that she and I would come down and listen. We got there for the last hour on Saturday night and realized Parker was very upset with the piano player. People were requesting tunes that Parker was associated with on his string albums, things like "Dancing in the Dark" and "April in Paris." But the piano player didn't know any of the tunes. Parker was giving the piano player a bad time, and the poor pianist, who happened to be a friend of ours, was very embarrassed. Suddenly Parker looked down and saw Lorraine and said, "Lorraine, would you come up here and sit in, please?" Lorraine agreed and Parker asked her if she knew "Stella by Starlight." People had been requesting it all night. Lorraine said she knew the tune. She asked what key and they went on with "Stella by Starlight." Lorraine played a solo, then Bird played. At the end of the tune, Charlie went up to the microphone and in that bravado style of his said, "Only once in a lifetime do we hear such great talent." He introduced Lorraine and then insisted that she play a solo with his rhythm section. While Lorraine was playing, Bird came down to me and led me by the elbow onto the bandstand. He put a chair by the piano and said, "Now you sit here next to your wife." It was so embarrassing, and then he whispered in my ear. "Now I know why you married her, because she plays all the right harmonies."[19]

Bird was right about that. Those albums that the Gellers made in the mid fifties for the EmArcy label are living proof that her harmonics brought out the best in her husband. The psychic interplay between Herb's alto saxophone and Lorraine's piano brings to mind Paul Desmond and Dave Brubeck or early Lee Konitz and Lennie Tristano, an intuition that occurs only after years of playing together.

Unfortunately, Geller's only LP as a leader, called *Lorraine*, is out of print. Here is the definitive Geller. Everything you ought to know about her piano style is showcased; her wit and rumbling left hand, the double-jointed phrases, and a ball-bearing, straight-ahead drive that lifts you right out of your seat. A better name for this album would have been *Intensity*.

In 1957, the Gellers bought a home in the Hollywood Hills. Later that year, Lorraine became pregnant with her only child, Lisa. Except for a short stint with Kay Starr in Las Vegas, she virtually gave up the piano after the baby was born. Jeannie Hackett thinks this was the happiest period in her life: "I visited Lorraine not long after the baby was born. The Gellers had a lovely home overlooking the city. She was thrilled with the whole thing. She and Herb had an ideal relationship. They were mad about each other and now she was a mother. I remember her saying, 'This is the most wonderful thing that's ever happened to me. I never thought I would be a mother.' Lorraine was not glamorous at all, she was large boned, had angular features and wore thick

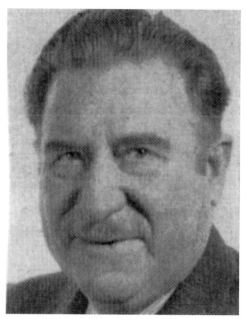

Wally Hanna (courtesy of Bob Trowbridge)

glasses. I think she figured early on that she'd never have a husband and a family."[20]

Herb Geller remembers the complex that Lorraine had about her appearance. "I remember she said to me once when she was looking in the mirror: 'My eyes are right; my ears are right, my nose and my mouth, but put them together and they don't spell mother.' Of course, I loved the way she looked." Her last appearance was with the Bill Holman Quintet on Saturday, October 4, at the 1958 Monterey Jazz Festival. A week later Geller's body was found lying next to her baby's crib, the victim of a fatal lung infection.

For a while the Acme was a learning center for six whiz kids, all from Fort Vancouver High School and all under the direction of Wally Hanna, a roly-poly wavy-haired music teacher with a touch of Richard Dreyfus's Mr. Holland. He

changed Bonnie Addleman from a violinist with the Portland Junior Symphony to a first-class jazz bass player. Later she put on a tuxedo and went on the road with Ada Leonard and her all-female orchestra. She moved to New York and joined the Roy Eldridge Quartet. She played for Tommy Dorsey, where she met her first husband, Ray Wetzel, who was killed in a car accident. Some of her best playing is with the Beryl Booker Trio on an early Discovery album. Her overall ambition, she told a *Down Beat* reporter, was to have an all-woman trio with Lorraine Geller on piano.[21] She credited a Jimmie Lunceford record for getting her started in jazz. That and Quentin Anderson's harmonic sophistication.

If it had been his style, Quentin C. Anderson, from Hanna's stageband, could have dropped names with the best of them. The lightly built trombonist played with or arranged for such jazz luminaries as Woody Herman, Billie Holiday, Georgie Auld, and Bill Evans. Originally from Minnesota, Anderson moved to Vancouver in the forties. While learning about music in Hanna's stage band, Anderson was also serving his apprenticeship at the Acme Club, playing with the Charlie Merritt Group, with Dick Knight on tenor and Lee Rockey on drums. The piano player was an early bopper named Kenny Bryan. After graduation Anderson made one of the best decisions of his life. He married his high school sweetheart Anne, a union that lasted a lifetime. They moved back to Minnesota to attend the College of Music. From there he went on the road

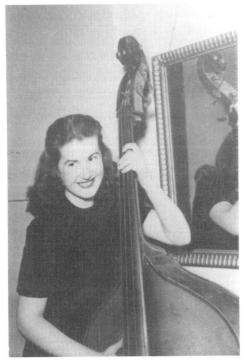

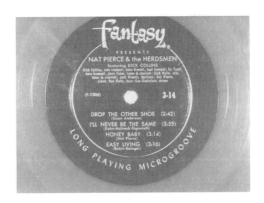

Bonnie Addleman Wetzel (courtesy of Lee Rockey)

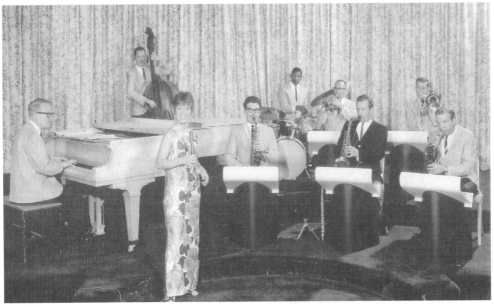

Quen Anderson with the Carl Smith Orchestra. Left to right: Bobby Dyke, Jerry Magill, vocalist Patti Hart, Earle Minor, Ken Johnson, Howard Gatley, leader Carl Smith, Quen Anderson, Braley Brown (courtesy of Carl Smith)

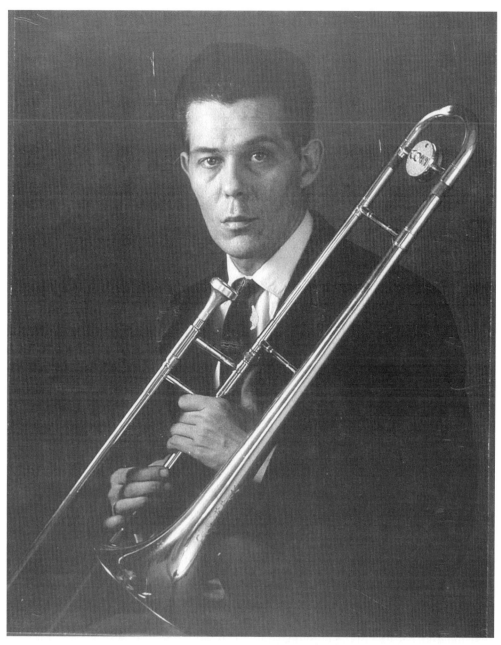

Quen Anderson (courtesy of George Reinmiller)

with bop singer Anita O'Day's all-star group that included trumpeter Don Fagerquist and the innovative drummer and composer Tiny Kahn.[22]

After moving to New York in the early fifties, Anderson joined the semi-sweet band of Charlie Spivak, where he sat next to one of the major stylists of the jazz trombone, Jimmy Knepper. When Knepper came through Oregon in the early eighties with the Charlie Mingus Dynasty, he and Anderson spent an evening reminiscing about those grand old days on the Midwestern band tour with the Spivak band. After his time with Spivak, Anderson joined Herbie Fields, who was fronting a sextet featuring a young and then unknown piano player by the name of Bill Evans. He and Evans developed a close relationship that was to last until Evans's death in 1980. During his time with Fields, Anderson also played with other big names such as Serge Chaloff, Frank Rosolino, and Billie Holiday, for whom he wrote several arrangements. Anderson left Herbie Fields in Philadelphia and moved to Los Angeles and not long after that was substituting for the great trombone player Ray Sims in the Dave Pell Octet, his most challenging assignment, he remembered, because of the ensemble voicings and the high caliber sidemen of that small group out of the Les Brown Band. Anderson also wrote a very swinging chart for Woody Herman called "After Theater Jump" and four tunes for a splinter group out of the Herman Band. Those arrangements and compositions make up the greater part of an album

released in 1954 on Fantasy Records by Nat Pierce and the Herdsmen.

Joining swing-era saxophonist Georgie Auld was his most satisfying stint as a sideman, although Anderson said he would just as soon forget the only record he made with Auld: a tribute to Perez Prado, the mambo king, on one side of a 45 rpm and a nod to Bill Haley and the Comets on the other. When Auld left New York in the late fifties, Anderson moved back to Vancouver, Washington, and began to write and play for an experimental jazz orchestra under the direction of Jim Smith and Ernie Hood. They performed in a club under the Hawthorne Bridge appropriately called the Way Out. It was there that Anderson had the unusual opportunity to play behind San Francisco poet Kenneth Rexroth in an attempt to wed poetry and jazz. In the mid-sixties Anderson spent most of his time writing and arranging for Freddie Keller and for the Carl Smith band. It wasn't just Patti Hart's vocals, or the great drumming of Nick Gefroh and Ken Johnson, or even the fine alto saxophone of Earle Minor that elevated Smith's band from good to great.[23] Mostly it was the arrangements of Quen Anderson, those same arrangements he had written for Nat Pierce and the Herdsmen. "Drop the Other Shoe," "I'll Never Be the Same," and "The King" launched the Carl Smith band. Smith and his band are still going, under the title of The Natural Gas Company, and Anderson's arrangements, some of them now forty years old, are still in the book.[24]

Personal problems forced Quen Anderson to put his pen and horn away for the major part of the 1970s. He returned in 1978, playing and writing for an octet called Bopsided. Just before the quartet's debut at Artquake in 1981, Anderson sat down for a newspaper interview and was asked what got him into jazz.

Two records, "Lester Blows Again" and Jack Jenney's "Stardust." Vic Dickinson plays on the Lester record. He was one of my strongest influences when I started. I remembered copying his solos on "Lester Blows Again" note by note, one bar at a time on manuscript paper, from an old 78 rpm Aladdin record. Jack Jenney's solo on "Stardust" is one of the greatest trombone solos ever. He was way ahead of his time when he recorded that in the late thirties. That solo has been speaking for itself for years. You know Jenney never showed off his technique like some players do today. What amazes me is that this record is as great today as when it came out. I wonder how many soloists today will last that long.[25]

Sitting in the saxophone section of many of the big bands in Portland in the forties and fifties was a tall, bored-looking blond who at a certain distance in a certain light you might mistake for a leading man in a "B" movie. Band leaders put up with his quirks, eccentricities, and well-known weak bladder because Dick Knight had a sound on the saxophone that still evokes a sigh twenty years after his death. It was a sound that formed in the bottom of his stomach, wound its way up his windpipe and out the bell of

his horn like a sultry tradewind. Every other tenor player on the Avenue was listening to Lester Young or Illinois Jacquet or Wardell Gray. Knight's man was the father, Coleman Hawkins. Knight also learned from Portlander Ralph Rosenlund, whose vibrant Ben Websterish tone and modest demeanor he admired. There aren't any commercial recordings of Dick Knight, just an on-location acetate done at the Acme Club in 1946 with Charlie Merritt and featuring Kenny Bryan, the often-mentioned transitional piano player who came to Portland from the Floyd Ray band and was one of the first to experiment with modern harmonies. The poor fidelity does a gross injustice to Knight's rhapsodic tone but he swings like mad, because he is fresh off a trip to Los Angeles where he played with Duke

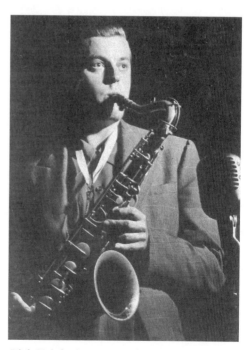

Dick Knight (courtesy of Colleen Knight and Lee Rockey)

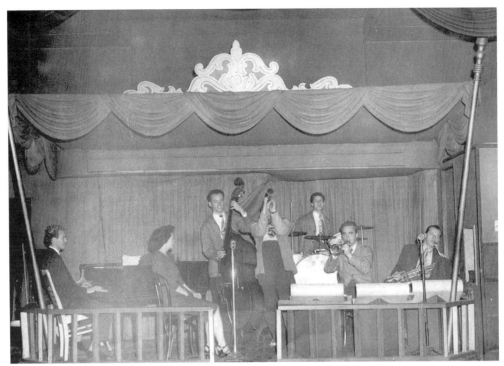

Dick Knight with Barney Bigard

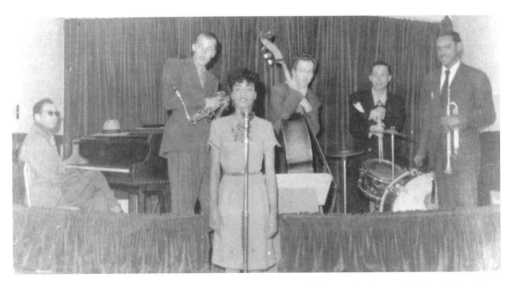

Dick Knight at the Acme. Left to right: Ken Bryan, Dick, Marie Bryan, Keith Hodgson, Lee Rockey, Charlie Merritt (leader)

(All photographs on this page courtesy of Colleen Knight and Lee Rockey)

Ellington's clarinetist Barney Bigard, an engagement that may well have been the high point of his musical career.[26]

Dick's favorite local big band was that of Earl Horn, for whom he wrote most of the arrangements. Horn was Earl Hornstein, owner of the swank King's Closet clothing store on SW Broadway. With the help of Ernie Hood, he realized a childhood fantasy by owning his own jazz band and filling it with Portland's top jazz musicians, augmented with some of the heavyweights from Los Angeles such as Lucky Thompson. The few 78 rpm recordings made in 1946 at the Bungalow in Seaside show a band ahead of schedule.

Knight also played with the fine Freddie Keller band at Jantzen Beach. Keller would take the microphone and announce a solo on "Stardust" by Richard Knight, and then Knight would play "Body and Soul." In the middle of the drum solo, he might hop over the band rail, run to the restroom, return to his chair in similar fashion and proceed as if nothing ever happened.[27]

Ernie Hood was a good friend of Dick Knight and when Knight passed away, he wrote this intimate epitaph:

He was a private person; only a few people were afforded a view of him. He was a man whose sensitivities were finely tuned, but he was nevertheless totally absent of sophistication. He played with some fine musicians: Sid Porter, Julian Henson, and jam sessions in downtown Los Angeles with Max Roach and Charlie Mingus. Yet he bore no haughty airs nor could he tolerate anyone who did.

Richard played loose, organic, warm, and ferocious; he had the strength of a bull and the gentleness of a pussycat. It was always a thrill for this pale skinny kid to pick up his tenor, lick his whistle, and terrify the socks off us. He once referred to himself as a ballroom slugger. Then he became disillusioned with life in the sixties. He spent most every day at home wearing his zoot suit pajamas. When he went to work at night sweeping floors and cleaning latrines for the Evergreen School District, he would dress in old cord pants and a blue work shirt, his uniform. His abstract paintings expressed the thoughts of riotous colors and spheres and were on display in the Vancouver Library, where he was the main janitor, a job he rather liked. Richard was unable to deal with everyday civilities but he communicated well with the Earth and its smaller creatures. He enticed birds to come and spend moments with him. Richard made us laugh so much. But he laughed much more than any of us. He may not have achieved success in the common world but his graphic expressability, his lifelong romance with his wife Colleen, and that two-week gig at the Plantation Club with Joe Turner made him a very rich man. [28]

There was even more talent in Hanna's stageband—Norma Carson, for instance, whose father got her started on trumpet. Hanna and Dick Knight took it from there. "I was inspired by a wonderful music conductor, Wally Hanna, and the whole city of Vancouver was behind him, getting us money so that our concert band could go on tour."[29] With Knight leading the way to the Acme or its satellite, the Chicken Coop, she listened to and reluctantly played with a raft of trumpeters equal to any in the history of Portland jazz. They were everywhere: Julian "Jay" Dreyer, Doc Severinsen, whom she competed against in high school, Skeeter Evans from the Art Roland Band, who was beginning to experiment with some of Dizzy Gillespie's ideas. Ben Roberts was around. So were Walter Bridges, Jack Dozier, and Bob Hibbler. Russ Hackett was playing at the Paddock. The smooth Don Proctor was at the Clover Club. Jimmy Lott was at the Rose City Club arranging jam sessions just before leaving to play with the great Jimmie Lunceford. And no one should ever forget the inventive Bobby Baker, one of the

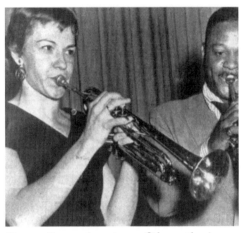

Norma Carson (courtesy of the author)

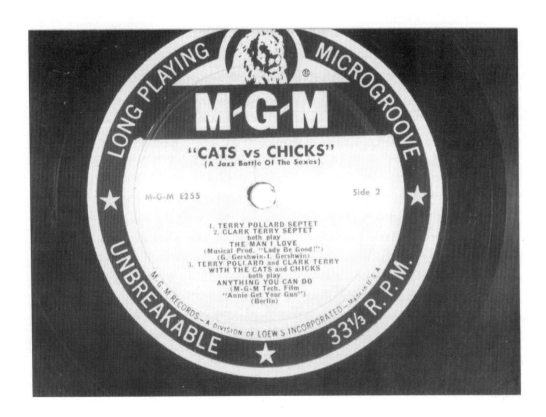

early white boppers, nor the short-lived brilliance of Don Norlander with Woody Hite.

When Fran Shirley left Ada Leonard's band to go with Charlie Barnet, she called Carson in Portland and asked her to take her place as the lead trumpet player. "I never thought about taking a jazz solo, but when I arrived, Ada Leonard said 'Norma you're going to have to play some jazz,' and I said, 'Oh no. I can't do that.' And I remember the first night I stood up and tried to play, I was so scared my knees were knocking. But what I hated most was having to wear the pink dresses with ruffles running all the way down to the floor."[30] When she left the band, Carson headed for 52nd Street in New York to play with the biggest names in jazz: Art Blakey at Birdland with her soulmate from Vancouver High School, Bonnie Addleman Wetzel, on bass. Reviewers called her the flaming-haired trumpeter from Birdland. But actually the crowd was ready to sneer her off the stage. She told Leonard Feather in her interview with *Down Beat* that "I never found it an advantage to be a woman playing jazz, 'cause some guys, like one tenor saxophonist with Jazz at the Phil, resented me." With the help of Oscar Pettiford and Billy Taylor she won the crowd over with her version of "Talk of the Town."[31] Her favorite place for a jam session was in the basement of the William Henry Hotel on Broadway, New York. Lorraine and Herb Geller would frequently drop in, along with dozens of other aspiring boppers. Everyone was learning from the same man, Charlie

"Yardbird" Parker. One of those early-morning sessions at the hotel came out in the late seventies on Zim Records, called *Charlie Parker, the Apartment Session*. Carson and her husband-to-be, Bob Newman, a tenor saxophonist, are listed on the back of the album as participants.

One night at the Cafe Society in downtown New York, Leonard Feather was in the audience again. In his column in the following issue of *Down Beat*, he compared Carson to the great Fats Navarro with the headline, "This chick plays like Navarro," and then Feather, a fierce supporter of women in jazz, set up a battle of the sexes between some very formidable female fireballs in New York and some of the best-known men musicians. It came out as a ten-inch LP called *Cats vs. Chicks*. "I was terrified, let me tell you, 'cause there were some very very good people on that record: Lucky Thompson, Clark Terry. We did a thing together called 'I Can Do Anything Better Than You' where we challenged the men." Carson loses the trumpet tiff with Clark Terry, but plays very well accompanied by Wetzel, on "The Man I Love."

Carson married Newman in 1952 and they started a family. She learned that her career as a fulltime jazz person was about to end. She felt grateful for as much as she had had, but there are some regrets.

I never had near as much playing in jam sessions as I would have liked to because that is where you really get to know your horn and the chord changes. That is what

gives you the experience. You can know every tune and every chord change but unless you experiment with it with other people in jam sessions you are never going to know what you can do. Listening to records gives you a lot of experience. You might not be an innovator like Bird or may not arrive at your own way entirely, but you are more apt to arrive at your own way of playing from hearing a lot of people on records. I never wanted to be an imitator but maybe there is some flavor of somebody you have been influenced by more than others. For me it was Clifford Brown; but that's what makes a good jazz player, when you can have a lot of different influences and still be able to play with that flavor and have your own sound. You know when you have played well. You know deep inside what you are capable of beyond what anybody else can say or what anybody else could write.[32]

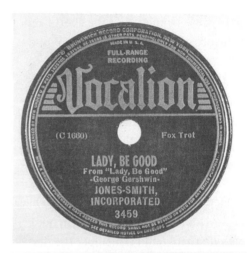

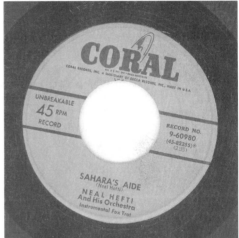

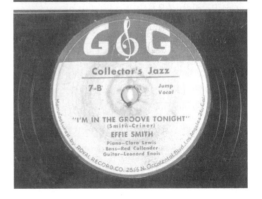

Another musician in Wally Hanna's school for swingers was Keith Hodgson, a bass player and a regular at the Acme before he went on to hold a chair in the revered Washington DC Opera orchestra. Fresh out of high school and looking younger, Hodgson was one of the few bass players in the area who had comfortably adjusted to the role of the bass violin in modern jazz. He studied his instrument like a scientist and looked to drummer Lee Rockey for inspiration.

Modern drumming in Portland starts with Lee Rockey, an unstudied, introverted Elvin Jones type. The intricate cross rhythms of rebop were as natural to him as breathing. Rockey, however,

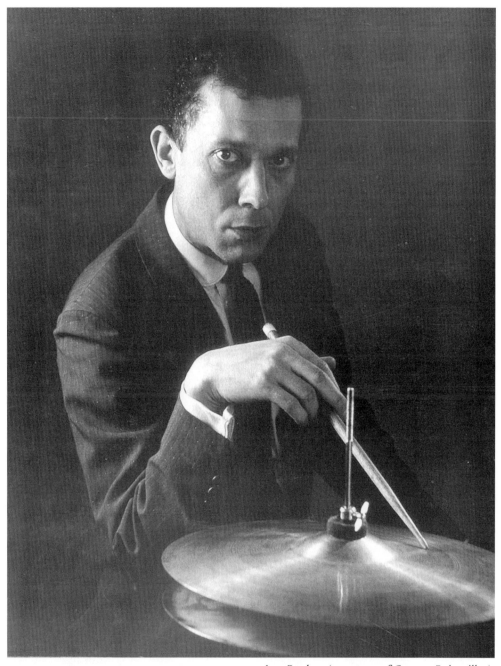

Lee Rockey (courtesy of George Reinmiller)

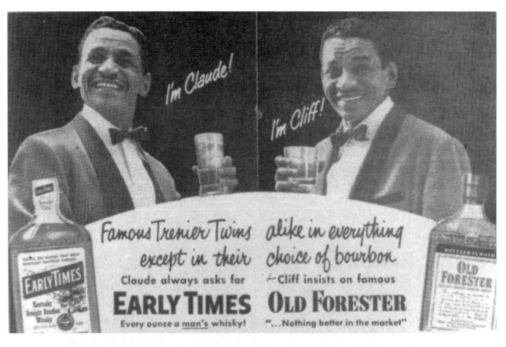

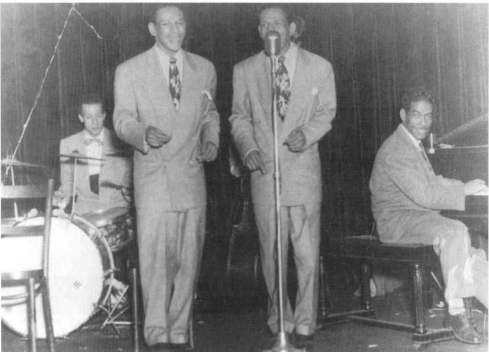

Lee Rockey with the Trenier twins and unknown pianist

(All photographs on this page courtesy of Lee Rockey)

was more interested in his early discoveries than what Hanna was saying in the music room of Vancouver High School. They were small discoveries at first, such as making a miniature drum kit with his Tinker toys. Then he found some old pots and pans and began to beat on them. And then one day in the back room of a barbershop, he and Dick Knight uncovered an old 78 rpm record of Count Basie playing "Lady Be Good" with Lester Young and Jo Jones. That really started things. The way Gene Krupa looked in the movie *Ball of Fire* in 1941 with Gary Cooper and Barbara Stanwyck reaffirmed his conviction to become a jazz drummer. "I couldn't get over the scene where Krupa plays a drum solo on a match box with little match sticks."[33] Rockey picked up more than a few helpful hints from the rudimentally sound Joe Amato, a symphonic percussionist and circus drummer. "He was just beautiful to watch," said Rockey.

In the mid forties, Rockey was backing up the Trenier twins at the Acme and driving Carl Thomas's Frantic Five at the Subway Grill underneath the Broadway Bridge. He was sitting in with Sid Porter at the Chicken Coop and holding down the drum chair as the only male in Hazel Fisher's big orchestra. Bonnie Wetzel was on bass. "Bonnie and I did our best and once in a while all the girls and I would actually get the beat going. But it was a hard push. There was Hazel, a large woman sitting at the piano in that sparkling burgundy dress, counting off Ellington's 'A Train.' It would seem like days before we could get it out of the station because she could never get the

tempo quite right, and before long the whole thing was like a train wreck," says Rockey. Eventually he went to New York and in 1952 he joined arranger Neal Hefti, who had a popular record out at the time called "Coral Reef." *Down Beat* did a full-page photo story showing a picture of Rockey and other members of the Hefti band. Hefti was one of the best arrangers in jazz and his wife, Frances Wayne, was a singer with a big hit called "Happiness is a Thing Called Joe." "It was all promise and no punch," says Rockey. "Neal had the guys and the arrangements but he would never pull them out and let us blow. Frances and Neal wanted something more commercial." Rockey's drums can be heard on one Coral recording of "Sahara's Aide," a spoof on "Scheherazade."[34]

In December of 1954 Rockey and his high school buddy Keith Hodgson and one member from the Hefti band were the rhythm section on Herbie Mann's first album. One track, a slow funky blues called "Purple Grotto," became the theme song for Al "Jazzbeau" Collins, a very popular disc jockey at that time in New York. Rockey returned to Portland in time to join Ernie Hood and Jim Smith's experimental orchestra at the Way Out, a Bohemian nonalcoholic jazz club under the Hawthorne Bridge. Hood, Quen Anderson, and Bill Hood did most of the writing for this all-star Portland group that included Lee Reinoehl, Dan Mason, Bud Gerlach, and—fresh from the Big Apple—Lee Rockey.

In 1964 he was part of the Jerry Magill Chamber Jazz Ensemble. After that he was a member of Jim Smith's Bossa Nova group. In the seventies he joined Lee Reinoehl and his seventeen-piece Stan Kenton-inspired concert orchestra. In the late seventies he teamed up with the organist, Count Dutch.

Sometime in the mid eighties, Lee Rockey sold his Mel Lewis style Cadillac green and gold Gretsch drums and took up the jazz violin. He became very interested in free music and preferred to leave bebop to his favorite disc jockey, KBOO's Don Manning. Lee Rockey died around Christmastime in 2002. According to his wife, his last request was a CD player and a copy of Count Basie's "Lady Be Good," the record that began his whole career.[35]

The favorite female vocalist among the regulars at the Acme Club was the former star of *Hell's a Poppin'*, Effie Smith. The management knew that it would be a profitable two weeks whenever they

were able to book her, which was often. Every jukebox up and down the Avenue had a copy of "Effie's Blues" backed up by the Red Callender Trio, but other than that and her 1944 arrangement of "St. Louis Blues" with Erskine Hawkins, there is very little of Effie Smith on record.

The reviewer of the *People's Observer* exploded with enthusiasm after seeing Effie's performance at the Acme. "Miss Effie Smith surprised everyone with her mad vocals. The mad song styling of this artist penetrates the consciousness of many of her listeners as a rocket bomb would in a haystack. Only with more impact."[36] In 1950 she returned, this time with a piano player who would make Portland his home and play a big role in the history of jazz in Portland, Warren Bracken.

Those at the Acme who liked their music on the party side got ready for the

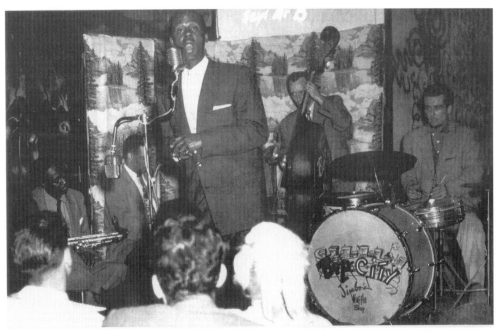

Saunders King at Jimbo's Bop City (courtesy of Carol Chamberlain)

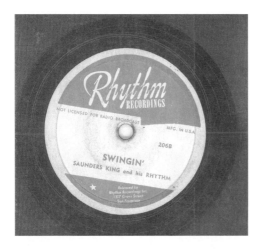

Trenier twins, Cliff, Claude, and their band of pranksters. This was a six-man vaudeville show combining vocals, tap dancing, tumbling, jazz solos, and a lot of nonsense. It was choreographed jump performed at a pitch near madness. The saxophonist would pretend to pass out from holding one note for almost two minutes, and the audience would cheer and howl while other members of the band tried to revive the actor with smelling salts. Later on, the Treniers became a big item, endorsing whiskey ads and making records for Decca.

Saunders King was another now-forgotten blues artist guaranteed to sell out at the Acme. His recording of "SK Blues," with the memorable line, "Put your fine mellow body on my knee," even outsold Effie Smith on the jukebox at Nance's Barbecue and at Bob Seeger's Victory Lunch. Jimmy Witherspoon made a record of it, so did Joe Turner and a number of others. You'd probably find it in the blues section of most record shops, but King's septet at the Acme was a jump group, blending riffs and bop figures from Dizzy Gillespie with electric guitar. Joe Williams of the Basie Band was one of many singers swayed by Saunders King. "He was a coal-black beautiful guy," says Williams, "whose lyrics and gut feelings I could understand and absorb."[37] It wasn't just on the Avenue where King drew big crowds; he was even more popular at Bop City in San Francisco, where he spent most of his time. He was the father of Sonny King, a leading alto saxophonist in the sixties and seventies. He was father-in-law to Nancy King, one of the few pure jazz singers from the Northwest.

CHAPTER 5

Lil' Sandy's

Saunders King, who played at the Acme, also liked to play at Lil' Sandy's, named after the son of its owner, John Tanaka. It was on the southeast corner of Weidler and Williams. They never booked any straight jazz acts because Sandy's was the center for the blues and a favorite after-hours spot of Big Mama Thornton, Little Esther, and once in a while, T-Bone Walker. T-Bone Walker, Charlie Christian, and Django Reinhardt represent the Holy Trinity of modern guitar. Walker pioneered the use of electric rather than acoustic guitar in blues combos. Jimi Hendrix, Bobby Bland, and Saunders King all come out of Walker's tradition. Walker once bragged that "he had a sound so unique that if two hundred guitar players were lined up each sounding a few chords by themselves, listeners would be able to pick him out of the crowd."[1]

Restaurateur Frank Nudo was there dozens of times in the mid fifties.

I'm not that big on instrumentals but I love singers, all kinds of singers. So when I got out of the service in 1956, somebody at the post office where I was working said I should go to Lil' Sandy's. On the outside it wasn't much, small neon sign saying dancing, cocktails. You entered at the side entrance as I

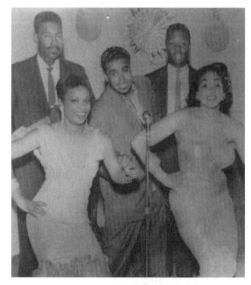

Left to right: unknown man, unknown woman, Eager Beaver, Chuck Moore, Cardella DeMilo (courtesy of James Benton)

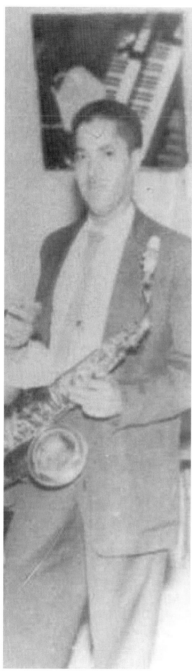

Sherman Thomas (courtesy of James Benton)

remember. There would never be any more than ten whites in the place and there would never be any problem. It was the safest place in town; any sign of a problem, the guy would be whisked out so fast it would make your head swim, like in the movies. There was never any cover at Sandy's and on Sunday nights when nobody else was doing any business, the place would be jam-packed. I used to see the boss there, big Tom Johnson, who owned many of the buildings in the area. When I opened Nick's Coney Island in 1960, he would come in for a coney and a glass of milk. I saw all the greats in Washington DC when I was in the service: Dinah Washington, Sarah, Ella Fitzgerald, but Cardella DeMilo at Sandy's with Chuck Moore on drums was all of them rolled into one. You name it, she sang it. All the great Ruth Brown tunes: "Work With Me Annie," "Oh What a Dream."[2]

Ralph Black had an equally spirited following and a voice the size of his six-foot-six-inch frame. In the parlance of hip, he had "heavy pipes." His favorite singer was Joe Williams and his favorite song was "Everyday I Have the Blues," that and a lady killer version of "The Nearness of You."[3] His only commercial recording is as guest vocalist on a Billy Larkin album for World Pacific done in the 1960s.

The happenings at Lil' Sandy's were rarely advertised. Folks discovered the week's venue from word of mouth or from Eager Beaver, an early Black broadcaster who conducted his popular

R&B radio show from the store-front window of the Melody Record Shop at 2713 N. Williams.

"We did fine with the blues but what really helped us," says Tanaka, "was the jukebox and the bottle law we had at that time. We counted on those as much as the live acts. Say you had a bottle of scotch. We would take it from you at the door and then make you buy our own mixer. Then we'd use your own liquor, basically charging you twice for the same drink, but all we did was sell you the mixer. Jukebox was a big money maker too, since we split the money fifty-fifty with the distributor. Most places had a jukebox in to make money. The quality of the music didn't mean all that much. At Slaughter's pool hall it was different, money came second."[4]

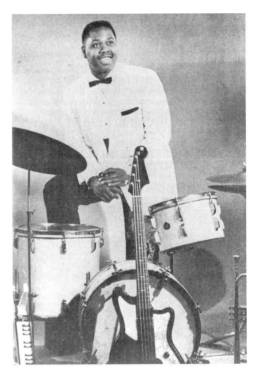

Chuck Moore (courtesy of James Benton)

CHAPTER 6

Slaughter on Williams Avenue

Below the Acme was the Savoy Billiard Parlor, a pool hall where you could find the proprietor, Ed Slaughter, jazz historian and honorary mayor of Williams Avenue. Slaughter was a thick-lensed, three-hundred-pound Good Samaritan, who probably lived his whole life without making a single enemy. It didn't seem to matter who you were, some prostitute or an ex-politician on the skids. If you were down on your luck, Slaughter would see you through, most of the time without interest or collateral. Drummer and blues singer Sweet Baby James Benton remembers Slaughter as the hippest guy in town. "He was like a great bartender in the know. The guy you always wanted to get tight with." Out-of-town musicians speak of him in the present tense, as though he were still presiding over those pool sharks who used to circle the tables when serious money was floating around, when Fast Eddy Collins and Willie Vance were squaring off and the place was packed, hushed, tempers edgy, like in *The Hustler* with Paul Newman.[1]

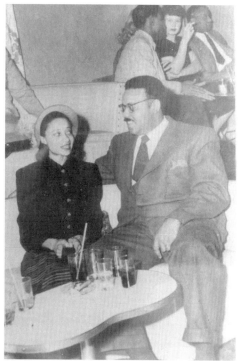

Bernice and Ed Slaughter (courtesy of Bernice Slaughter)

Black children in the public schools were learning next to nothing about their own history. At the Savoy Billiards, Slaughter was telling stories about Duke Ellington, Count Basie, Roy Eldridge. "We used to gather 'round him and he'd tell us stories about Lester Young and Louis Armstrong," says former city commissioner, turned disc jockey and jazz writer, Dick Bogle. "He had a big bass voice, and with his knowledge of jazz, he would have made the best disc jockey, but there weren't any jobs for Blacks in Portland in those days." Bogle was reviewing records for the *Portland Challenger* in 1952. The name of his column was "Slaughter on Williams Avenue" because the jazz records being reviewed were the ones in Slaughter's jukebox. "You could blindfold me, send me back sixty years, put me on the

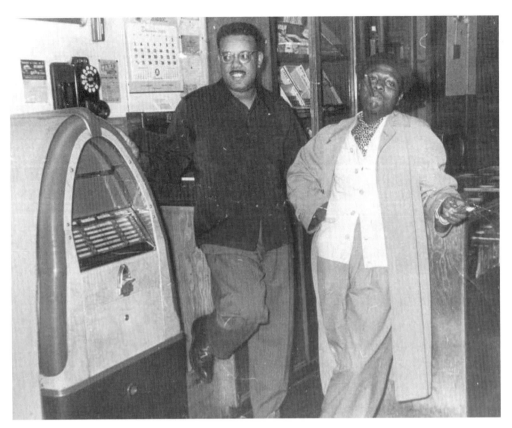

Ed Slaughter and the Canned Ham, with an unidentified admirer (courtesy of Bernice Slaughter)

"The Best Juke Box in Portland"

SAVOY BIILIARD PARLOR

1508 N. Williams Ave.   VE 9104

corner of Cherry Court and Williams, and I'd still know exactly where I was because of the smell of the barbecue and the sound of the jukebox."[2] Jukeboxes were everywhere, all up and down the Avenue, in soda fountains, churches, schools, nightclubs, diners, dance halls, even gas stations and drycleaners had one or more of these nickel-hungry entertainment centers. In ethnic neighborhoods and Black communities where there were few record players and no radio stations playing their music, the jukebox was everything.[3] "We didn't have no players, no radios, the jukebox brought us the music," says blues singer Jimmy Witherspoon.

More popular than the pool tables, or even Slaughter himself, was his jukebox, aptly called the Canned Ham for its resemblance to a Hormel ham tin. It was no top of the line model, had no neon whirlygigs, no layers of gingerbread and whipped cream. It was a Pontiac in the hierarchy of jukeboxes, manufactured in Kansas City where Ed Slaughter himself came from. Like most jukeboxes, it came equipped with a two-ton tone arm and a steel needle capable of grinding a 78 rpm record into white powder in less than fifty plays. Slaughter's selection of jazz and blues records inside that jukebox was a reflection of his infallible taste, born out of years in one of the major cities of jazz, Kansas City, at a time when his own step-brother, Merle, was playing tenor saxophone with the immortal Charlie Parker.[4] Merle's name is mentioned in the liner notes of a Charlie Parker album as having been the one who introduced Charlie Parker to

Norman Granz and his Jazz at the Philharmonic.

As far as anyone knows, Slaughter never learned to play a lick. Instead he was a jazz messenger, spreading the music and its stories wherever he went. More than a few future jazz musicians heard their first record on the Canned Ham. Benny Goodman, Artie Shaw, and occasionally Duke Ellington were on network radio. If you wanted to hear James Moody's "Mood for Love" or Private Cecil Gant's "I Wonder," two of the best-selling records on the Avenue, then you had to go to the pool hall.

"I heard a Billy Eckstine record on Slaughter's jukebox and decided right then and there I was going to practice harder," says Cleve Williams. Williams is from Hope, Arkansas, a house just down the street from his cousin and alter ego, Bobby Bradford. It's within walking distance of where former President Bill Clinton lived. If you were a child in Hope, you took music in school even if all you ended up doing was pounding the top of a Quaker Oats box. "You will notice that Clinton plays the saxophone," says Williams. "That's what I wanted to play, but the other kids beat me to it, and I ended up with the only instrument left, the baritone horn. I didn't like it at first, but thanks to a teacher named Jimmy Cannon, I won a state contest with it. That was the same year that Bobby won on trumpet."[5]

Both of their parents came to Portland to work in the shipyards in 1942. When Williams got here, he gave up the trombone for a while to become a singer in the Billy Eckstine tradition. Eckstine

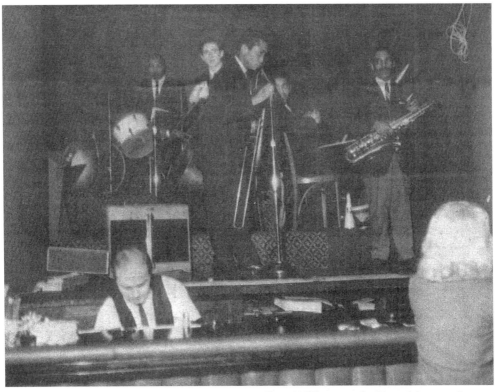

Cleve Williams at the Terpsichorean Room
at the Park Haviland Hotel. With Williams:
Bobby Bradford, Bob Mabane, Evans Porter,
and Dave Weinstein. In the foreground,
bartender Duane Rohlffs. (Courtesy of Cleve
Williams)

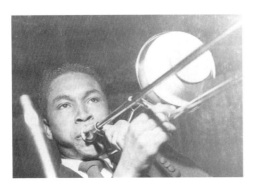

Cleve Williams (courtesy of Cleve Williams)

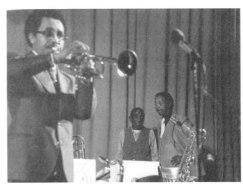

Bobby Bradford (courtesy of Joanne
Hasbrouck)

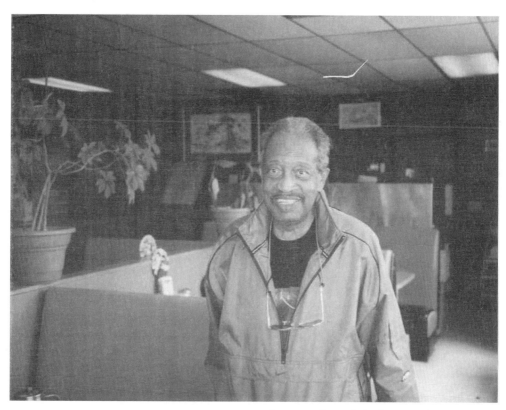

A recent shot of Al Johnson, who played bass at Jackie's (courtesy of Ron Weber)

was also a very good trombone player. " 'Everything I Have is Yours' was my favorite of his," says Williams. It was one of the songs he sang when he opened for Billie Holiday at the Civic Auditorium in 1949. "As I was getting off the stage, soaked with sweat from being so nervous, she whispered as she passed by, 'Very nice, young man.' " Williams's only recording under his own name is a vocal on the Modern label, last seen some forty years ago. "My idol in town was Mel Brown's father-in-law, Eric 'The Voice' Boyce. He was very much in the Billy Eckstine manner."

Bradford went into the service and came back full of this new thing called rebop: Dizzy Gillespie, J.J. Johnson,

records he'd heard while he was stationed in the Philippines. For Williams's birthday, Bradford got him a trombone, and then they both started playing in the Herb Amerson band out of Vanport. They played at the Frat Hall, and also the Oasis and at the Vanport Recreation Center before the big flood of 1948. It was a Black band with a white drummer, who, according to Amerson, was very good. However, it was confusing to one of the guests at an Elks dance in southern Oregon who walked up to the stage during intermission and asked Amerson when their regular drummer would be coming back.

Jackie's Cafe is where Cleve Williams, Bobby Bradford, Roy Jackson, Les

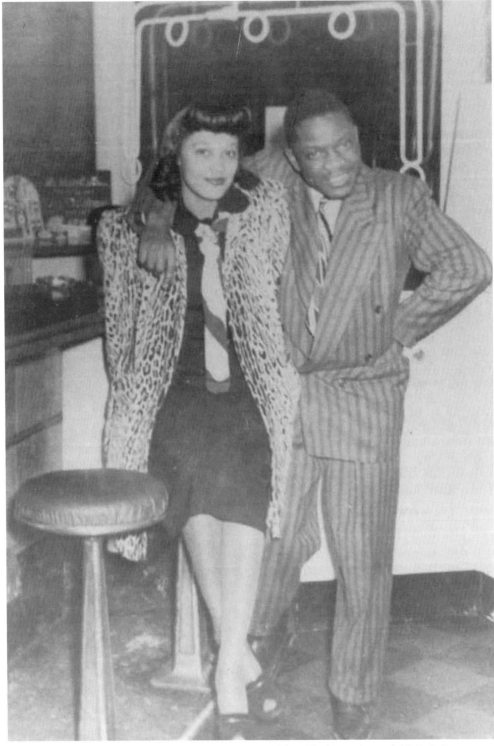

*Unidentified couple at Jackie's Cafe
(courtesy of Bob Williams)*

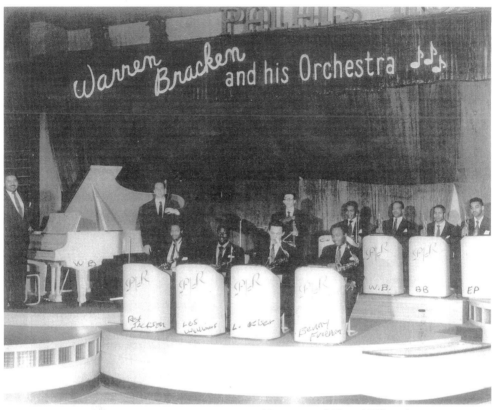

(Courtesy of Cleve Williams)

Williams, and trumpeter/pianist Evans Porter learned to play. It was on the corner of Weidler and Victoria, about where the Sherwin-Williams paint store used to be. Like most of the buildings in the area, it was owned by Tom Johnson, and like the Coop and Paul's Paradise it was an after-hours joint, where the local heroes gave the youngsters lessons. In 1949 the whole Count Basie band showed up, making it one of the most exciting evenings in Williams's young life. "They were hanging out the windows," Williams says. And then there was the night that Gene Ammons came in from Jantzen Beach and played "More Moon" to a packed audience. Later, novelty band leader Kay Kyser brought a group of fresh-out-of-college sidemen into

Jackie's, peach fuzz and all. They had finished their dance engagement at Jantzen Beach and came looking for Williams, Jackson, and Bradford. "They were huntin' us down," says Al Johnson, the bass player, "they were huntin' us down like animals. We laughed at them at first, and then they started in, and the only one who could keep up with them was Les Williams. Of course, Les was playing his ass off in those days. It was humiliating. I still don't know who they were. But it's that competition that made us get better. You have to know what's out there."[6]

Williams was drafted into the Army Signal Corps during the Korean conflict. A certain godsend lieutenant, a personal friend of bop trombonist J. J. Johnson,

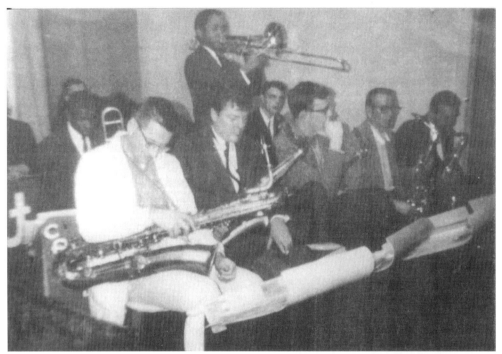

Cleve Williams (standing) with the Walter Bridges saxophone section, left to right: Bill Hood, Dick Knight, Ron Hite, unknown, Braley Brown (courtesy of Cleve Williams)

saw to it that Williams was transferred to the corps band. "I often wondered what happened to him. He probably saved my life, and most definitely influenced my career," says Williams. "I think of him a lot and wonder if he is still alive." His Army band had some of the most talented players in the United States. One of them was Richard Boone, an ex-Count Basie sideman. He helped Cleve with his technique. "And then playing eight hours a day at parades, reviews, and dances, you can't help but get better," says Williams, "especially with a guy like Richard Boone showing you the way."

Williams returned to Portland and refined his newly acquired craft in the forgotten Warren Bracken big band. One night Dinah Washington came into

McClendon's Rhythm Room and hired Porter, Les Williams, Jackson, and Williams right off the stage. She took them to Los Angeles, where they stayed with Redd Foxx, the comedian, who was also a jazz enthusiast. Washington, in the meantime, went about augmenting Portland's best with some of L.A.'s finest: including Frank Morgan, Addison Farmer, Teddy Edwards, and Jimmy Cobb of the Miles Davis band. "Oh, it was the absolute highlight of my life," says Williams. "She took us on a tour all over the West, but before we could make any records with this all-star group, she left for New York. Before she left, she gave me a picture. I still have it and she signed it, 'You sure can play the blues, Cleve. Dinah.'

"Dinah helped me make some records with Jimmy Witherspoon. He called me 'Homeboy' because he's from a town about the size of Troutdale, thirty miles away from Hope. Roy Jackson got some solos on all four of the records we made on the Federal label for Ralph Bass."

When Williams got back to Portland, he joined the best of the many editions of the Walter Bridges big band. Bobby Bradford took most of the solos, but the real feature was the saxophones: Dick Knight, Bill Hood, Braley Brown, and the wonderful Ron Hite, who Williams remembers as "another Marshall Royal." Hite hung up his horn soon after to become a celebrated high school teacher at Sherwood and later Oregon City, where for a while a large portrait of him hung in the main entrance. His career was the subject of a short-lived network TV series starring David Hartman.

Toward the end of his career as a full-time jazz musician, Williams teamed up with Bob Mabane, a tenor player and roommate of Charlie Parker when they were together on the Jay McShann band. Williams found him in Montana and coaxed him into coming to Portland. Eventually Mabane found a job as a baggage handler at the Portland International Airport while becoming a regular member of the Walter Bridges big band, where his big number was "Deep Purple."[7]

Williams hasn't played regularly since the mid-sixties. Every once in a while when the spirit of J. C. Higginbotham moves him or his soulmate Bobby Bradford prods him, he'll reach down from his La-Z-Boy chair, unlatch the case that holds his burnished horn, squirt on some slide oil, put his lips to the mouthpiece and, in the words of the great Warren Bracken, "He do what he do, singin' the blues on the slide trombone."

Bobby Bradford and Cleve Williams are spoken of in the plural like Bob and Ray, the comedy team. They went to the University of Portland together. They still live close to each other, and two of the few times they were separated were when they were both in the service and when Williams went to Los Angeles with Dinah Washington. Washington wanted Bradford too, but he wouldn't travel. His priorities are unaltered: faith, family, music, in that order. According to Williams, he has had offers from Earl Bostic and Charlie Barnet, who liked his playing so much that he had him flown to Las Vegas for a weekend date; and when Illinois Jacquet and his brother got into a fight at the Ozark Nightclub in 1953, Bradford was asked to replace him. Bradford's first hero way back in Hope, Arkansas, was a former Erskine Hawkins trumpeter who lived only a couple of doors down. On their way to school, Williams and Bradford would stand and listen to the half-valve techniques and the lip slurs of this ex-trumpeter named Brigham. He took young Bradford under his wing and within a short time, he was one of the top trumpeters in the state.

At Slaughter's pool hall, he heard Charlie Parker's "Now's the Time," a B-flat blues featuring a young Miles Davis on trumpet. Davis's soft attack and understated ideas appealed to Bradford's own quiet, unassuming manner. Bradford never seems to have a bad day. He can be in a noisy jam session standing next to musicians he has never played with, some of whom have had too much to drink, and still come up with something, like the chorus he took on "Misty" at Braley Brown's bacchanalian memorial. "Like a nightingale in a foundry," quipped one onlooker.[8]

In his seventies he is still playing well, as a recent CD by the Albina Arts Ensemble attests. The drummer on that date is Chris Conrad, one of the many drummers in town who is grateful to be in Williams's and Bradford's presence. "They were like godfathers to us," says Mel Brown. "They gave me my start at an Elks Club dance one day." And the high-profiled Ron Steen says the duo gave him his first job at the Doubletree Inn. "They are unsung heros," says Steen. "Every time I play with these cats, someone comes up to the bandstand and says, 'Where did they come from? How long have they been in town?' Oh, a little over fifty years. Where have you been?" asks Steen.[9]

Slaughter's jukebox also helped along the career of little-known Walter Barney Benton. For eight formative months between his junior and senior years in high school, Benton divided his time between sitting in at the Frat Hall, playing fullback for Benson High School, and plugging nickels in Slaughter's Canned Ham for one more listen to Count Basie's "Avenue C" with Lucky Thompson. There are traces of Lucky Thompson in Benton's only record as a leader. Riverside Records went all out and hired Miles Davis's rhythm section

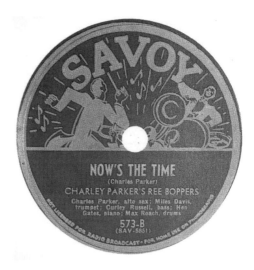

plus Freddie Hubbard. *Out of this World* was the album's title and Benton's "virile all man" tenor earned him four stars in *Down Beat*.[10] He was in faster company a few years earlier with the Clifford Brown all-stars featuring Max Roach. In the sixties Benton made several records with Max Roach and then disappeared.

Bill Hilliard, the former editor of the *Oregonian*, roomed with Benton during the time he was here in 1947. "I can still hear him practicing, getting ready to go out to play, and he would still be in his Benson High School marching band outfit. He was an overgrown, plump, happy-go-lucky kid with a jumbo-sized talent to go along with it. I lost track of him for awhile, and then when I was in L.A., I saw him for the last time, sitting on a cot in jail. He'd gotten into drugs, and one leg had been amputated. But that happy-go-lucky attitude was still there."[11]

CHAPTER 7

Jumpin' at the Record Shop

All you had to do to get one of those hits on Slaughter's Canned Ham was walk up Williams to Broadway. On the southwest corner was a faded red and beige building about the size of a tennis court. A large plate glass window said "Records for sale"; letters above the door said "Madrona." It was a manger compared to the CD supermarkets of today. Stacks of records sat on wobbly tables. There were makeshift bins and dusty shelves stuffed with albums and hard-to-get blues and jazz singles. On the top were stand-up cardboard displays of famous recording artists. There were two glass-enclosed listening booths with turntables and enough room for mambo addicts to work out. There was a cash register, a counter, another record player, and that was about it.[1] Not the kind of place you would expect people to be talking about fifty some years later. But Madrona was more than just the only place in town to buy Black music, called race records then. It was a social center and a meeting place, a twentieth-century version of an eighteenth-century coffee house abuzz with the latest platter

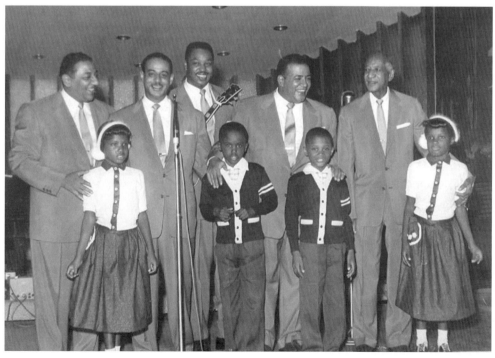

The Mills Brothers with Portland's first set of quadruplets (courtesy of Amato family)

chatter. It was a hangout for hep cats and a place where new musicians in town could find out about job opportunities. "Hang out there long enough," says blues singer James Benton, "and you are likely to run into Joe Louis or Paul Robeson. I practically lived there for a while. I met the Mills Brothers there with Joan Crawford and that fat cat from the *Checkmate* TV show, Sebastian Cabot."[2] Charley Garrett, one of the most important figures in the commercial development of Williams Avenue, opened the store in 1938, just when phonographs were making a comeback from the Depression.[3]

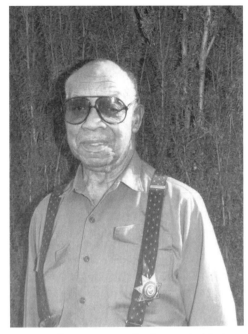

Fay Gordly (courtesy of Bob Trowbridge)

Ed Slaughter had a secret source for acquiring the records in his jukebox. Charlie Garrett depended on hip waiters and porters from the railroad for his weekly supply of race records from Chicago and New York and Los Angeles. Fay Gordly was a porter with the Union Pacific Railroad in the forties. "When I had enough seniority, I got the forty-hour one-way run to Chicago, and Charlie Garrett knew it and also knew that I was a jazz fan," recalls Gordly. "So one day he comes up to me and says, 'Hey fella, how about picking up these records I have on my list here, and you can keep a couple for yourself.' Well, I had a portable phonograph like many of the guys I was working with on the railroad, so I'd fill my suitcase full of Jimmy Rushings and Jimmie Luncefords in Chicago, and then I would get to keep some for my efforts; but of course porters were bringing in more than just records: booze, gage, anything that was hard to get, choice steaks."[4]

Madrona Records was a magnet for music lovers from all over. One was Bill Haseltine, the foremost authority on Stan Kenton in Portland. A long-time resident of the West Hills, Haseltine is sure he would never have visited the "other side" were it not for the treasures that lay buried in those beat-up crates in the back of Madrona. "I went over there in high school because they had the Charlie Parker Dials that I had read about in *Down Beat*. I ended up there regularly for a while because of a jazz album put out by Norman Granz called *Jazz Scene*. It was the most expensive thing in the store, black glossy cover, gold lettering. Inside were photos by a famous photographer. It sat on a high pedestal behind the counter. I couldn't get the thing off my mind. I still remember the look on the clerk's face when I told him I was going to buy it."[5]

Another West Hills traveler to Madrona was the former state senator Ted Hallock. In his youth Hallock was a Peabody Award-winning disc jockey and the first *Down Beat* writer from this area. Later he wrote for the British *Melody Maker,* thus bringing the activities of Williams Avenue and elsewhere in Portland to the attention of an international audience. By that time Charlie Garrett was long gone, and Al Grant, pianist Tom Grant's father, had purchased the store.

After I got to know him a little, I'd go into the store and say, "Hey Al, what's new," and he'd usually say "Nothing," and I'd say "Don't give me that crap," and he would go behind the counter and *come back with some Prestige, some Blue Notes, some Savoys for me to play on my "Spins and Needles" radio show, stuff you couldn't get from the main distributor.*

Al was a reed-thin chain smoker, with a slick sense of humor that mixed sarcasm with wit. He always had a tan like he just got off the plane from Miami Beach. I was telling people on my show on the Westside to go to the Eastside for the best jazz and swing records, even though I remember having a small apprehension myself about the Avenue in those days. But the Avenue was very safe. I saw a lot of musicians there, Pat George, that fine trumpeter Jay [Julian] Dreyer, a lot of white-ass cats who went there because I told them to. My Madrona plugs on the air were so good that I was MGM's disc jockey of the month.[6]

Hallock started his music career as a neophyte drummer in Pat Riley's Grant High School stage band. He had no technique, no formal instruction, but made up for it with plenty of flair and a thirty-inch bass drum with a nude Lady of the Lake on the front, illuminated by a fifty-watt lightbulb inside. "You'd like looking at it," says Hallock, "even if you didn't like my playing." Hallock improved by sitting in at the Cherokee Club, a place that was one floor below street level on SW Park Avenue between Alder and Washington. The band leader there was Bob Hibbler, a Black trumpet player who later joined Jimmie Lunceford. "He was very nice to the young players who were trying to

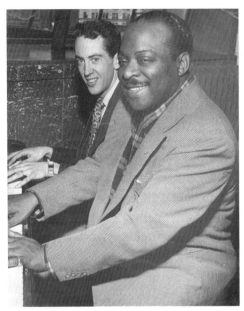

Ted Hallock and Count Basie (courtesy of Ted Hallock)

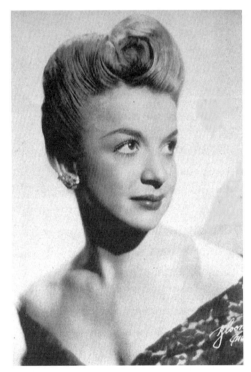

Trumpet star Frances Shirley (courtesy of Margaret Havlicek and Phil Hunt)

establish a reputation by letting us sit in. He wore three-inch-high tab collar shirts that were just magnificent. Of course in those days I had my own zoot suit made at Ralph Grabler with a knee-length coat, pants up to the armpits, a gold key chain, a high-neck shirt. That was my uniform. Norm Thompson [the clothing retailer] owned the Cherokee Club. Food was a myth there, booze was your problem," says Hallock. "Oregon was against liquor by the drink in those days. You brought a pint or a fifth in a brown paper bag. You peeled the top of the sack back and sucked it, or you gave it to the bartender to serve you and charge you for your own liquor."

Before going into the Air Force, Ted Hallock started having jam sessions on his late-night radio program, which in those days was recorded on the seventh floor of one of Portland's landmarks, now the PGE Building. Ernie Hood was often on guitar, Dick Knight on tenor, Fran Shirley, the trumpet player, was there. Marty Wright played the alto saxophone, and on piano was John Merriman, a future math professor at Notre Dame. "I played drums," says Hallock, "and then one night Lee Rockey shows up. I hated Lee Rockey. I was considered good until he started playing."

After the war Ted Hallock went to the University of Oregon, where he put together a fine band. The recording genius Wally Heider was the baritone saxophonist. Ted Hallock began writing for *Down Beat* in the late forties. It was Hallock who did the first story on another regular at Madrona Records, Sammy Davis, Jr. It appeared in the July

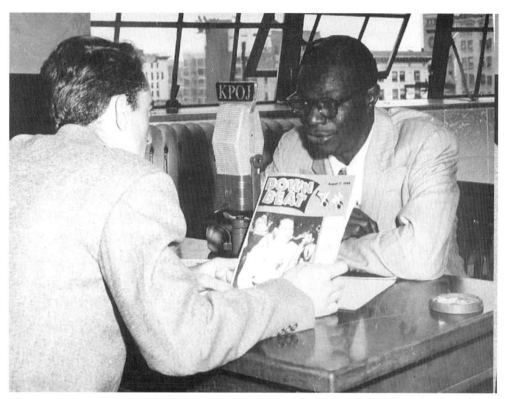

Ted Hallock interviewing Nat King Cole for his "Spins and Needles" radio program (courtesy of Ted Hallock)

1950 issue of *Down Beat* under the title "Sammy Davis and How He Grew." Hallock's main point was that Sammy Davis was so versatile, so talented in so many areas that he couldn't make up his mind what he wanted to do. "If you heard him sing 'The Way You Look Tonight,' " says Hallock, "you'd know that nobody, but nobody, could imitate Frankie Laine, Nat King Cole, and Billy Eckstine the way Sammy can."

Sammy Davis, Jr. was in Portland frequently in the late forties and early fifties as part of the Will Mastin Trio, playing at the Civic Auditorium or at Amato's swank supper club, or at the Clover Club, which was across the street from where the Central Library is. When

he finished his act, Sammy Davis, Jr. would head for the Clarion, under the Broadway Bridge, where he enjoyed playing with trumpeter/pianist Russ Hackett. Davis, by day, was often seen rummaging through the bebop bins at Madrona Records, carefully placing each newly purchased Charlie Parker record in a leather briefcase that never left his sight.[7]

"On the way up, he was on the Avenue for some time," says Bill Hilliard, "and was not popular with many Blacks because he was playing clubs downtown where Blacks were not welcome."

In an interview with writer John Wendeborn years later, Sammy Davis acknowledged his apprenticeship in

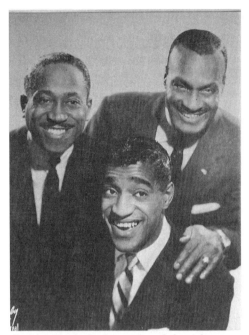

Sammy Davis, Jr. (center) and the other two members of the Will Mastin Trio at Amato's supper club (courtesy of Margaret Havlicek and Phil Hunt)

Portland, especially the tap dancing routines by the legendary Teddy Hale, another daily visitor to Madrona Records when he was in town. Teddy Hale was not the kind of person who would confine his dancing to nightclubs or the vaudeville stage. He might start dancing at any time, anywhere. At the drop of a needle he could turn Madrona Records into a theatrical set, stopping the buyers in their tracks with his off-the-wall choreography. This went on in people's living rooms, too. Bernie Slaughter tells this story: "Ed and I used to have him over and we'd put on his favorite record, 'Exactly Like You,' and he'd be dancin' all over the house, jumping over the furniture, flying out of the bedrooms, doing a slide across the kitchen floor. He couldn't stop himself."[8]

Hale came to Portland as part of a Black vaudeville revue where he was billed as "Ted Lewis's shadow," referring to the movie roles he had had when he was five years old mimicking in miniature the great entertainer's every move. At ten he had been part of a dancing act with Ethel Waters, and by the mid-forties he was playing the Paramount in New York and the Apollo in Harlem.[9] Greater than Bojangles? If you believe what those people who saw him at the Acme had to say. A Gene Krupa in taps, or as Ed Beach put it, "a stand-up Buddy Rich." "He was able to do more with his feet than most drummers can do with their hands," says Clarence Williams. "Jazz drummers used to come in every night just to pick up new figures. He was the best this city ever had." When tap dancing went the way of the drop kick, Teddy Hale fell into

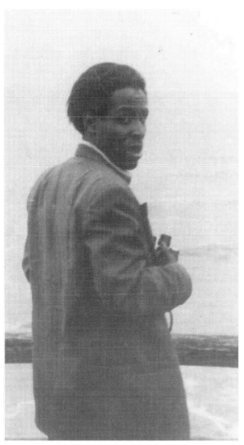

Teddy Hale at Ecola State Park, 1947 (courtesy of Bernice Slaughter)

an abyss of drug-filled days. He was working as a janitor in Washington DC when he died of an overdose at thirty-two.

Kenny Hing, from Tigard High School, who went on to take the great Jimmy Forrest's chair in the Count Basie band, got part of his inspiration from the enlightened selection at Madrona Records. "I memorized that album Stan Getz did," says Hing, "the one that had 'Stars Fell on Alabama,' 'Body and Soul,' and 'Nice Work if You Can Get It.' I wore it out. Before that I wanted to be Benny Goodman. I can still play 'Why Don't you Do Right,' the one with Peggy Lee. It's still beneath my fingers sixty years later. I could go to the horn right now and play it flawlessly. I was practicing thirty hours a week when I started taking from Eddie Flenner in the sixth grade. If it's saxophone you wanted to learn, Eddie was the man. You basically lived with your instrument. You practiced and practiced and listened and listened until you got enough confidence that you didn't freak out under pressure."[10]

Other musical inspirations for Hing were Sid Porter, Dick Knight, Ralph Rosenlund, and certainly George Lawson, the great might-have-been, who used to drop into Madrona Records. Lawson was into bop before anyone, and was coming into Madrona listening to the latest bop stars. "Why, he was so far ahead of me I couldn't believe it," says Hing. "I wasn't soloing that much or even playing that much jazz. I was working in the dance bands of Johnny Reitz and Dick Schwary and Bill Becker. And then I was going to Jantzen Beach and getting knocked out

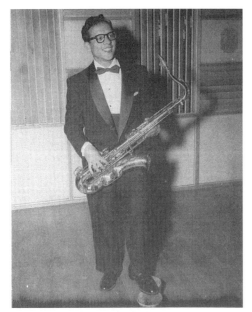

(Courtesy of Virginia Black)

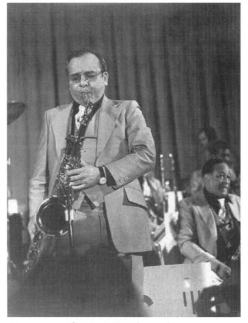

(Courtesy of Joanne Hasbrouck)

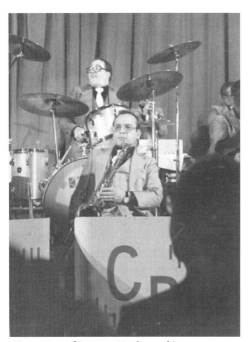

(Courtesy of Joanne Hasbrouck)

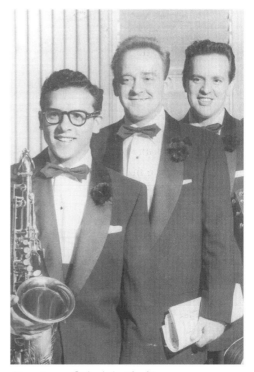

(Courtesy of Virginia Black)

Kenny Hing, clockwise from top left: as a teenager; taking a solo with the Count Basie band; with Eddie Wied and Warren Black; with Duffy Jackson, drummer

by some of the bands they were bringing in like Les Brown of the mid-fifties, the one that had the arrangements by Frank Comstock. They just blew everybody away that night, made a big impression on the musicians who saw them."[11]

Kenny Hing went to Las Vegas in 1958. The casinos and shows paid good money, and everything on Williams Avenue was closing up anyway. One night at an after-hours place called the Tender Trap, a couple of Count Basie sidemen discovered Kenny Hing. They wanted to sign him up right away. "It's hard to believe but I almost didn't take the most prestigious chair in the jazz business. No one turns down Count Basie; but I had never been on the road before. I was forty-some years old and there was the fact that I never had really been a soloist, even though I played at the Tender Trap. Jimmy Forrest came up and asked me right on the spot if I would take his place. But I was reluctant. I didn't hear anything for about several months and then one day the manager of Count Basie called and said I was in the band. I didn't even have to audition. That was in 1977."[12]

In the eighties, Hing would return to Portland occasionally for a date with Woody Hite or to sit in with Neil Masson and Jean Ronne at the Benson Hotel or with like-minded Harry Gillgam at the New Market Theater. Those who attended the Jazz Society's 1984 First Jazz Party heard Gillgam and Hing at the peak of their inventiveness, made possible in part by the alert all-out swing of drummer Carlton Jackson and bassist Tim Gilson.[11] Kenny Hing's solos have been praised by trumpeter Thad Jones and by the Count himself, who called Hing the outstanding soloist on the *Farmer's Market Barbecue* album. Kenny's personal choice is the chorus he took on "All The Things You Are" from the Sarah Vaughan/Basie album.[12] In the late nineties, he produced his own CD called *Little King*, his nickname in the Basie band.

CHAPTER 8

Jumpin' at the Savoy

In the spring of 1947, the Acme became the Savoy. The new managers, Norm Resnick and Si Denton, opened with Ivie Anderson. She was the rage in Portland, going all the way back to the 1920s when she was reported to have been here with Sonny Clay's Plantation Orchestra from Los Angeles.[1] Anderson was Duke Ellington's featured vocalist when he first played in Portland in 1933. In 1937 she sang "All God's Children Got Rhythm" in a Marx Brothers film and her popularity soared. Asthma forced her to retire from the Ellington tour in 1942. After that she opened a successful restaurant in Los Angeles called the Chicken Shack. In the mid-forties she began coming to Portland four to five times a year,[2] usually at Amato's Supper Club or the Clover Club, where her favorite accompanist, Gene Confer, was playing. She liked his chord voicings and clever introductions.[3] She also liked playing with Phil Moore, another Portlander, who arranged and played piano on a set of 78 rpm records she made just before opening at the Savoy.

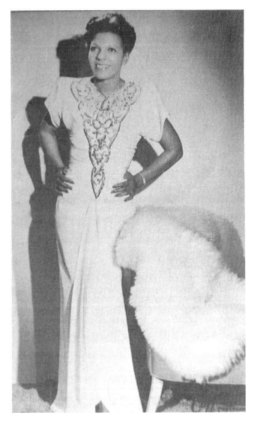

Ivie Anderson (courtesy of Margaret Havlicek and Phil Hunt)

An even bigger fan of Gene Confer was the still-active Eddie Wied, who started playing at the Savoy when he got out of the Navy in 1947. "I was living on Williams Avenue for a while," says Wied.

Nights I'd be playing either on the Avenue or with Freddie Keller's Orchestra at Jantzen Beach, sitting in along with Rod Levitt and my favorite saxophonist, Sam Schlichting, who I think was also living on the Avenue at that time. My days were spent sitting at the piano with some record I was trying to imitate, getting ready for the Avenue, to see if I could play that way in person. Williams was like a Harlem on the Willamette, everybody all dressed up. Hats were very big then. I even had a modified zoot suit. It was very friendly, very mixed and relaxed like when white people first went to Harlem in New York. If you heard somebody play, you'd want to keep up with them, even do better. The better the competition, the better you play. So I never looked at the cutting sessions as a cutthroat deal.

The Savoy, Paul's, and Jackie's, and other places on the Avenue are where we young players went to school. You can go to college now at Mt. Hood or Clackamas, but it's not quite the same as learning your trade on the Avenue or from one of my big influences, Sid Porter at the Coop. I remember Stan Kenton came into the Savoy one night. That was the first time I got to play with some heavies, so to speak. That must have been around 1948. Anyway, Shelly Manne was on the drums and there I was on piano, just nineteen years old.[4]

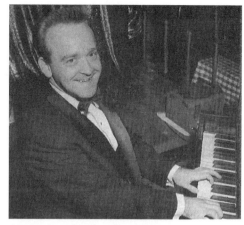

(Courtesy of Margaret Havlicek and Phil Hunt)

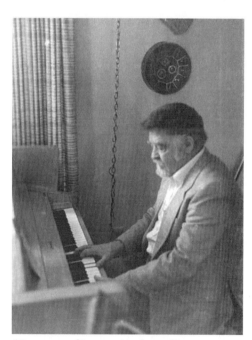

(Courtesy of Joanne Hasbrouck)

Eddie Wied, then and now

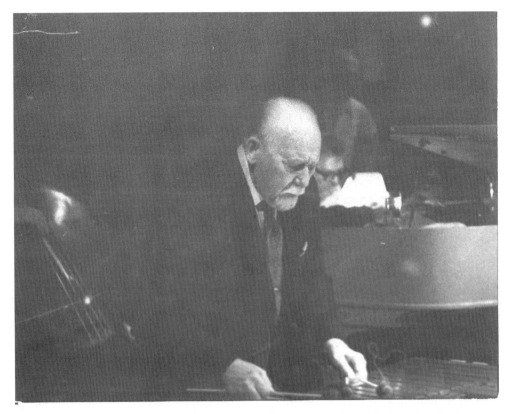

Red Norvo with Eddie Wied at the Jazz
Quarry (courtesy of Joanne Hasbrouck)

It was at the Savoy that Wied met up with Don Brassfield from Salem, who had been in and out of Portland for about ten years, spending most of World War II playing saxophone with Gene Krupa until the legendary Charlie Ventura replaced him. Brassfield was the featured soloist for Bob Crosby's swing to bop band when they played Jantzen Beach in December of 1945. In the early fifties, Brassfield had a club named the Blue Note, located on the Dallas Highway out of Salem. On Sundays, Cleve Williams, Bobby Bradford, Les Williams, and Wied would drive to Salem to play in the jam sessions conducted by Brassfield.

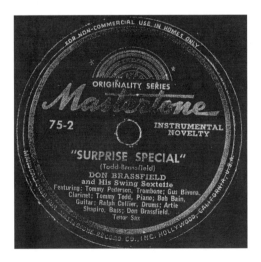

Ed Beach has a different take on Brassfield. He played with him in some nightclubs in Portland and remembers Brassfield as a tall odd-looking guy with glasses and enormous tone. "His big hit was 'Tico Tico,' " says Beach, "which he liked to play in the impossible key of B and when I couldn't make it, he really put me down. He threatened to beat me up. He finally forced me to quit." [5]

In 1951 Wied's picture was in *Down Beat* as the piano player with the Eddie Lawrence Quartet, a well-mannered group very popular at Jack and Jill's.[6] Eddie Wied moved to Las Vegas in the mid-fifties, where for fifteen years he was musical director and pianist for Tex Beneke and the Modernaires. His picture, along with the rest of the Beneke orchestra, is on the cover of a Warner Brothers LP titled *Something New*; Wied's featured number is "Baubles, Bangles, and Beads."

Since returning to Portland, Wied has rarely missed a day of piano work. He likes to say that "being a musician is a full-time job, like being a doctor. It just doesn't pay as well." He was the house pianist at the Hobbit in the eighties and earlier at the Jazz Quarry, where he backed up such well-known jazz artists as Red Norvo, Carl Fontana, and Jack Sheldon, who called him "the best in the Northwest."

One event Wied's fans might remember was when he, Mel Brown, and Leroy Vinnegar, a rhythm section that could swing a Shriners band, were the supporting cast for Georgie Auld at the Village Jazz in Lake Oswego. Auld was one of the big stars of the swing era, the point tenor man for Bunny Berigan, Artie Shaw, and Benny Goodman, with dozens of jazz albums to his credit. Just before they began the last set, Auld told a sold-out audience, "If I'm lying, I'm dying, but playing with these guys for the last three nights is not work at all. It is a ball. And I can't wait to come back, and in the meantime I think I'll take them with me."

Most of what they played that night was from the swing era. One of the exceptions was Johnny Mandel's "The Shadow of Your Smile." At the end of Wied's solo, Auld paused, looked at someone in the front row, leaned over and whispered, "Hey, what's going on here? They paid to see me."[7]

Wied spends most of the time teaching these days. One of his students was responsible for Wied visiting Italy not too long ago, out of which came a CD, appropriately called *Eddie Wied in Italy*. "I'm teaching now," says Wied, "because I saved all of my lessons and notes from Gene Confer, to whom my brother introduced me at about the time I was playing at the Savoy. Confer was my biggest influence. How could you not help sounding like Gene if you took lessons from him? The arrangements were irresistible. When I was playing in Las Vegas, Tex Beneke came up to me more than once and asked me who I studied with to get such lovely voicings. When I came back to Portland, I wanted to study with him again because I loved talking to him almost as much as the lesson itself. He inspired you. That is what a teacher is supposed to do, isn't it? Inspire you. All of us that studied with him, Harry Gillgam, Dick Blake, we all sound a little bit like him. That's really something, isn't it?"

Proof is in Dick Blake's lovely *How Deep is the Ocean* CD. "Besides all that technique I got from those two-handed exercises Gene used to write out for me," says Blake, "I learned about clarity, about how to get a certain sound out of the piano." Blake might well have had Gene Confer in mind one night at the Hobbit in 1987 when he started off the last set with "Polka Dots and Moonbeams," a song every student of Confer learned early on.

Harry Gillgam is a man of a thousand songs, an unerring ear, and a devotion to the Confer method. "Gene was the major influence on my career," says Gillgam. "I credit my progress to him. He loaded me up on drills and those great chord forms and turnarounds, which I in turn teach my students. But Gene was more than just a friend; he was like a father to me." Whether Gillgam is backing up an abstract altoist or revving up the rhythm section in Art Abrams's Swing Machine, he is comfortable in any setting, not the least of which was the trio he had at the Prima Donna, an intimate piano playhouse on SW Fourth, just around the corner from where Sidney's was. What Gillgam's fans soon discovered was that he could sing, really sing, with a rich perfectly tuned baritone voice, and a sense of phrasing apparently learned from Frank Sinatra records and from backing Nola Porter and the remarkable Ronny Gaines, Vancouver, Washington's, Mel Torme.

Confer's influence is so spread out by now that it is hard to imagine that at one time you couldn't walk into a piano lounge without hearing variations on Gene Confer. From 1938 until he died in 1981, he taught Jean Ronne, Tom Grant, Lorraine Geller, Warren Bracken, Bill McClendon, the talented Russ Hackett, and just about every other piano player in town, how to get beautiful music out of the piano. It seemed as though anyone with a good set of ears from symphony conductors to plumbers wanted a lesson from him. People used to joke that breaking into the Confer circle was as difficult as getting into West Point. Jean Ronne, the leader of one of the most successful quartets in recent history, was one of the lucky ones who got to study with him. "I got into jazz when I saw George Shearing," says Ronne, "but after a while I needed a left hand, and that is when I came to Gene. Without his guidance, I wouldn't be playing today. I can still see him standing in the doorway of his studio in the Fine Arts Building in that polo shirt he used to wear."

If you wanted to hear Confer play, you had to catch him when he wasn't aware, when he thought no one was listening outside his studio. Then out of the cracks and through the window shaft would come this relaxed, succinct, technically flawless style, a little like Buddy Cole, with whom he had studied in the Navy. Lush, intricately voiced chords steeped in the sounds of Ravel and Debussy became his trademark. They reflected the early training he had had with Dent Mowry, a dapper protégé of the great Claude Debussy. Dent Mowry has had more than a little influence on the evolution of jazz piano in Portland.

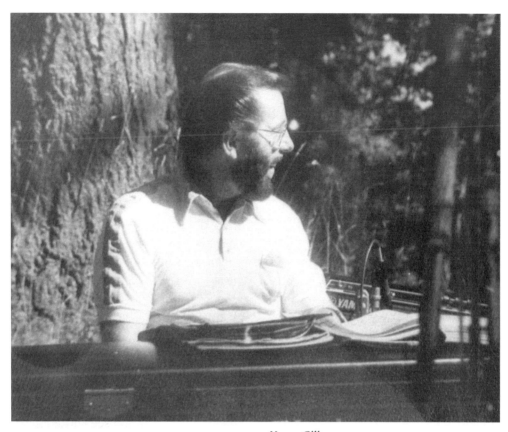

Harry Gillgam

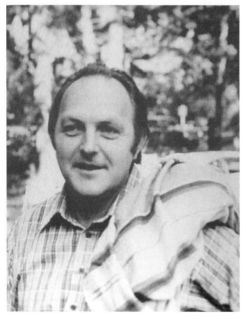

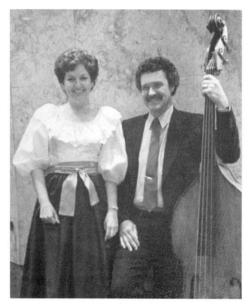

Jean Ronne and Fred Hard

Dick Blake

(All photographs on this page courtesy of Joanne Hasbrouck)

A lot of people never understood why Confer preferred teaching to performing, because in the forties he was one of the most complete piano players in town. "Sid Porter showed us how to swing," says Hallock, "and Confer showed us those beautifully voiced chords." Confer and Tommy Todd were among the first white modernists in Portland. As mentioned, it was at the Clover Club on SW Taylor where Confer made his reputation, backing up Ivie Anderson and other Ellingtonians like Ben Webster and Jimmy Blanton. He also played in back of Sammy Davis, Jr. One night Serge Chaloff, Woody Herman's poll-winning baritone saxophonist, dropped in. Those were the days of the floor shows, and the all-purpose Confer could sight read in a blackout. His best friend and band mate, trumpet player Don Proctor, remembers: "We were part of the Russ Graham Group. Sometimes we had Monte Ballou or Bill Hood. For a while it was kind of a crazy mix and whenever Gene would get excited, he would start wiggling his ears."

In the early fifties, Confer was at the keyboard at the Indochina Club on Barbur with the fine Hank Wales on bass and Artie Shaw's former tenor saxophonist, Ralph Rosenlund. "It was the best little group I've played with for flexibility and ease," says Rosenlund. "We never had any arrangements. Gene would just play one of those beautiful introductions and off we'd go." Wied, Gillgam, and Pat George would never miss an opportunity to hear him play in his days at the Clover. "We wanted a lot of notes," says Pat George. "All he

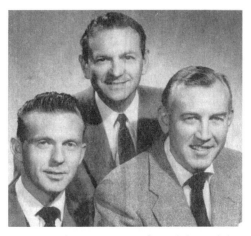

Gene Confer Jazz Trio. Left to right: Ralph Rosenlund (saxophone), Gene Confer (piano), Hank Wales (bass). (Courtesy of Ralph Rosenlund)

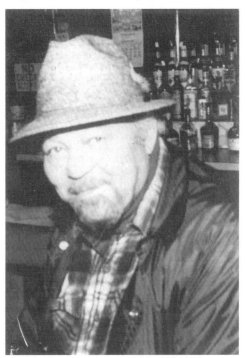

Julian Henson (courtesy of James Benton)

wanted was to get a beautiful sound out of the piano. He was a real perfectionist who never let his amazing technique interfere with his good taste, and no way would he ever fake a request like a lot of players I know do. If he didn't know the tune, he wouldn't play it, and no amount of money would change him either. I taught in the same studio in the Fine Arts Building for a while and when a student would cancel, he would practice a song like 'The Shadow of Your Smile' for a whole hour. He really hated mistakes."

"Perfection is the mark of a great player," Confer used to say. He never talked about himself. He really didn't care if anyone knew how great he was. He could have been a big-time studio player in Hollywood like Tommy Todd or Phil Moore, but he was happy teaching—and what a teacher.

Students would come to him not even able to find middle C, and about a week later they would be playing chord changes to "Ghost of a Chance." It was more like musical therapy than like piano lessons. You hung on his every word. You learned about Nat Cole, Bill Evans, and why the piano is the most satisfying instrument of them all. The self-effacing man with the Fred Astaire walk could lay a spell on you. He did on Tom Grant, for example, the son of the Madrona owner, who started playing at ten years old. "I came to Gene at my Dad's request, but he figured I was too young so I had to audition for him. I still remember the tunes. It was 'Laura' and 'Lullaby of Birdland.' Afterwards he looked at me and said, 'Hey, let's go for it.' I studied with him for five years."

Warren Bracken heard Confer play somewhere around the early fifties and he took several lessons, arriving at the opinion that if he had studied with Confer early on in his career, he would have had a lot more work in California before moving to Portland. Bracken said that Confer's sound on the piano was comparable to the sound that Dick Knight could get on a tenor saxophone.

A newspaper reporter and former student of Confer was one of the last to see him. He wrote this: "I remember walking into Gene's hospital room the day before he died. I was hoping to get my words just right, so I said, 'You have quite a legacy out there, you know.' He looked at me disapprovingly, motioned me forward, and in a dry limpid voice whispered, 'Bull.' "[8]

One pianist at the Savoy not affected by the Confer mystique was Julian Henson. Henson says, "Confer took one look at me and said, 'Sorry, but I can't do anything for you. It would only take away from your unique approach and your one-of-a-kind fingering.' I had musical parents, but my style really comes from an Art Tatum record made in the 1930s called *Sophisticated Lady*." Henson's other influence was Palmer Johnson, a Fats Waller-style pianist who was around Portland in the early thirties. Henson had his first piano job at sixteen, but he had no piano. So he found a church on North Larrabee Street that would allow him to practice and where he and a very young Sid Porter would trade new ideas, things they heard from Al Pierre or Don Anderson at the Frat Hall or possibly one of the bands coming up from California,

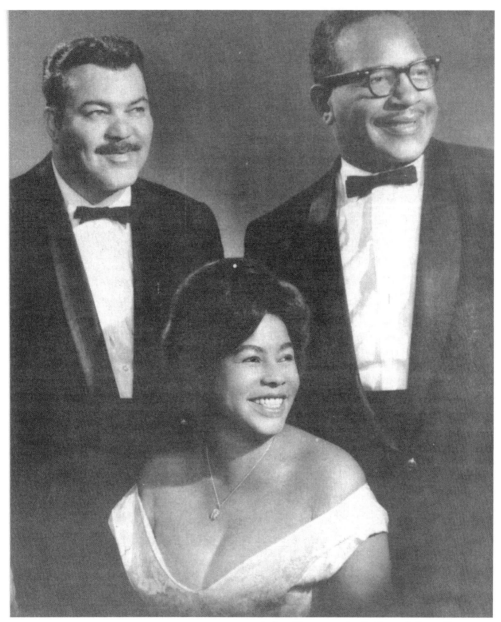

Julian Henson trio. Left to right: Julian Henson, Marianne Mayfield, Ira Mumford (courtesy of Robert Redfern)

like Curtis Mosby, in particular. Mosby and his Dixieland Blue Blowers were a twelve-piece orchestra featuring the future Ellington trombonist, Lawrence Brown, and future Count Basie altoist, Marshall Royal.[9]

Around 1932 Henson's father, a club car waiter, moved to Seattle. Julian Henson went with him and had a very successful career there. Paul de Barros, in his excellent book on Seattle jazz called *Jackson Street After Hours*, talks about Henson's influence on Jimmy Rowles, who at one point in his career spent some time in Seattle.[10] In the 1980s, Rowles was still calling Henson every month. Gerald Wiggins was another name piano player who spent quite a bit of time listening to the unknown Julian Henson when he was in Seattle. As early as 1945 Ed Slaughter was telling people in Portland about this Tatum-like piano player from Portland whom he had heard in Seattle. Henson moved back to Portland when the liquor laws made it tough on jazz musicians in Washington. He spent the rest of his life becoming the best unknown piano player in town.

Dale Harris played drums with Henson at Elmo's, a club way out on Sandy. "Compared to Sid Porter, Julian had to stretch just to reach tenths on the piano. But I think people will tell you that he was the closest thing to Art Tatum that this town has ever had. Funny thing is that nobody knows it outside a small circle of piano fans," says Harris.[11]

When jobs got scarce on the Avenue, Henson's fans followed him to Carmen's in the Hollywood District, where he played piano in a Las Vegas-like lounge

group called the Carmenaires. Solo space was limited to novelty ragtime numbers and eight-bar introductions to "Blue Velvet" and other hits of the day. In the mid-sixties he put a trio together with Ira Mumford on drums and marvelous Marianne Mayfield on bass. Mayfield came with impressive credentials. She was raised in Oakland among a bastion of blue-ribbon jazz talent that included Saunders King, Sonny King, and Carl Thomas, three names that would eventually be important parts of the Portland jazz story. On the way to Portland, she made an important stopover with the often-mentioned Big Jim Wynn and his Bobalibans, a backup group to T-Bone Walker.[12]

One of the places the Henson Trio played was the Pink Bucket tavern, a cement-block building painted passionate pink at SE 50th and Powell. The bartender would whistle along in tune with Henson's piano and the jukebox was limited to mostly Oscar Peterson 45s. Once each set Henson was able to stretch out on "Softly as in a Morning Sunrise" or the frequently requested "What's New."[13]

Occasionally he would sub for Sid Porter, who had his own club on SW Fifth and Lincoln. "We learned together as kids," said Henson, "so he would call me whenever he couldn't make it. I always admired his long fingers and relaxed style."

Henson still can't believe that he got fired from the Savoy for not playing enough blues. "Tatum rarely played the blues because everything you play in jazz has that atmosphere anyway. Well, I just took Basie Day and Clarence Williams, my whole group, and we just went across the river to the Circus Room. That's where they had us on the marquee on the outside of the club on a sign that read, 'Straight from Williams Avenue, acquired at great expense, the great Julian Henson featuring Portland's Prince of the Blues, Clarence Williams.' That still tickles me to this day."

Clarence Williams came to Portland to live for the same reason as Al Hickey, Julian Henson, and other Seattle musicians. Things were rotten in the state of Washington for jazz musicians. The reason was Bill 171, a law legalizing booze and wiping out the bottle clubs and after-hours places in one inky run of the governor's pen. "When things started to go bad," says Williams, "we'd finish our gig at the Washington Club or wherever, all jump into a car and drive 170 miles at 90 mph just to be somewhere that didn't close at one in the morning. And finally some of us just moved to Portland, Oregon. Hey man, it was the happening place in the late forties and very early fifties." Before moving to Seattle, Clarence Williams had been a big draw on Central Avenue in Los Angeles, backing up saxophonist Tom Archia at the Gaiety and Maxwell Davis at the Club Alabam. Williams was also leading a band that included saxophonist Jay McNeely. Later, when he was known as "Big Jay McNeely," king of the honkers and squealers, Williams was his guitar player, and supporting actor in McNeely's Theater of the Absurd. At concerts, teenagers went crazy when Big Jay would lie on his back screaming to the high

heavens, feet kicking in the air like some helpless insect while Clarence or some other member of the band stood over him with a microphone.

Williams made some records while he was in Los Angeles, some with Luke Jackson on the Modern label, records that have recently been made available on a CD set. Williams thinks he may be on a couple of records with McNeely, but he can't remember which ones. At the Savoy in Portland and at Lil' Sandy's down the street, he was billed as the Prince of the Blues, or better yet a hometown T-Bone Walker because he played the guitar and sang like him; he dressed like him; he danced like him; and had a preference for the same kind of Kansas City riffs and Texas longhorn blues.

Williams and sidekick Smiley Turner would do a takeoff on the Inkspots, starting with "I Didn't Know." And that's when it happened, an incident reminiscent of the 1999 film *Sweet and Lowdown,* where Sean Penn plays a Django Reinhardt worshiper who freezes in the presence of his master.

Savoy was always filled in '47 and '48 and I was just getting ready to sing when I looked up to see the man: Cab Calloway in Portland for a Porgy and Bess *show at the Civic Auditorium. You have no idea how big he was in the late forties, as big as Duke Ellington, maybe bigger. I froze. It really shook me. I panicked and stood there trembling, unable to move my fingers or my mouth. Cab sensed something so he came up to the stage and motioned me to come forward. Then*

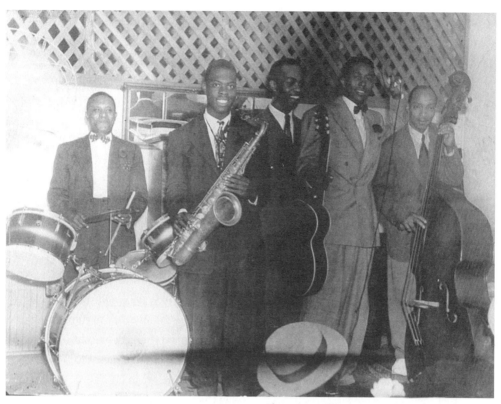

Clarence Williams (between guitar and bass) in Los Angeles, leading his Red Hot Band with Jay McNeely on tenor sax (courtesy of Clarence Williams)

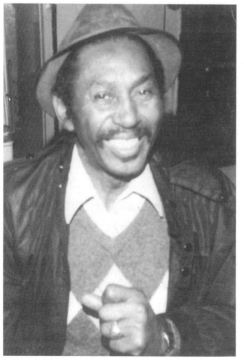

Clarence Williams (courtesy of James Benton)

he whispered in my ear, "Hey, man, sing your song, somebody will hear you." And it was like a balmy breeze washed over me and I completely relaxed. I'll never forget what he did for me that night.

Later on things started to change a little in Portland when the lady mayor, Dorothy McCullough Lee, took over. One night at the Savoy a couple of guys from City Hall came in and the next thing I knew, I was fired for singing dirty lyrics. Of course they were nothing compared to today's Grammy winners. I got the Los Angeles Union involved in this and they got me back my job at the Savoy, but what I later discovered was that the problem wasn't the lyrics but the little Jewish girl I was going with. That was the thing that was rubbing everybody the wrong way. Mixed couples in this city did not set well.[14]

In December of 1947, the Savoy brought back Big Jim Wynn. Like his protege, Big Jay McNeely, Wynn played bop and straight-ahead jazz for a while until he found he could make more money sprawling and squawking to the future generations of Elvis Presley fans.[15] Wynn named his sidemen, two of whom were the Trenier twins, the Bobalibans, because of a smash hit, "E-bob-a-leba." A favorite among the men at the Savoy was Jim Wynn's "The Shipyard Workers Blues," a macho plea for the return to prewar conditions, when women were back in the home.[16]

The single most important event at the Savoy in 1947 was the coming of Sonny Criss and Wardell Gray. They were in Portland for five months, according to Criss, but within weeks of their arrival it seemed that every saxophonist in the Northwest was coming under their domination. Legends in the making in your own backyard, on their way to the Hall of Fame. They came to the city in place of Billy Eckstine who had booked a tour of West Coast jazz cities but at the last minute was called away. So Eckstine put together a sextet featuring Criss and Gray and then picked Al Killian, the high-note trumpet champion, as leader. Killian was the leader, but Gray was the star.

What a year he was having. In February he was on a milestone recording session with Charlie Parker that produced the jazz classic, "Relaxin' at Camarillo." In April his solo, "Blue Lou," at a concert in Pasadena, California, was the record of the year in France. On July 12, he made "The Chase," a six-and-a-half-minute tenor battle with Dexter Gordon that was so popular on the jukebox at Slaughter's and at Madrona, and all over the country for that matter, that Dial Records could simply not keep up with the unexpected demand. Looking back more than half a century, it was Gray's best year.[17] Heroin had yet to turn his body against him. He could play all night without getting tired. He ate up competition like a piece of rare roast beef. Gray was not as original as John Coltrane or as important as Lester Young, but there were few who could top him in a saxophone battle. Portland's Warren Bracken would second that. He was on a Billy Eckstine record along with Sonny Criss and Wardell Gray made in May of 1947. Bracken and Gray remained friends long after Bracken had moved to

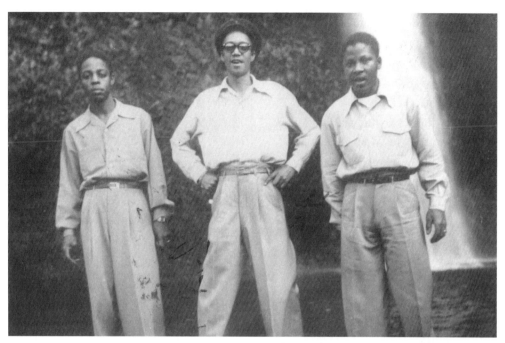

Left to right: Sonny Criss, Wardell Gray, and Tim Kennedy at Multnomah Falls (courtesy of Bernice Slaughter)

Portland. "He just liked the action, not knowing who he might run up against. He would stalk the after-hours places in any city we happened to be in, looking for a friendly duel, like some gunfighter in those Westerns on television."[18]

Gray's instinct for laying it on the line appealed to the crowd at the concert halls and at the Savoy where his nightly nemesis was Sonny Criss, one of the many sparring partners who brought out the best in Gray. Also there was Sonny Stitt at the Open Door in New York, with Jack Kerouac in the audience,[19] and of course Dexter Gordon, his most formidable opponent on "The Chase" and later "The Hunt." "The Hunt" was playing on the radio at a wild party in one of the episodes of Kerouac's *On the Road*: "To the sounds of Wardell Gray and Dexter Gordon blowing 'The Hunt,' Dean and I

played catch with Mary Lou over the couch."[20]

Kerouac had a tenor saxophone fetish. He went to see them in nightclubs; he wrote about them; he made records with them; and even imitated them in his ideas about spontaneous prose, the aesthetic for *On the Road*. His work is rooted in the purity of expression evident in the recordings of Brew Moore, Al Cohn, Wardell Gray. There is no stopping to pick the right word or musical note, no editing, no revision. The use of Gray's name in such an important book would have pleased him. He fashioned himself a worldly man. He was up on politics; he played chess; he read voraciously. When Ted Hallock interviewed Wardell Gray in the *Melody Maker*, he said this: "Interviewing Gray is more like attending a literary tea at

Aspen, Colorado, than interviewing a jazz event. Wardell would rather talk about James Michener, not about music. Of course he tosses in some jazz quotes once in a while but you have to work to get them, things like 'Bop is swinging,' or 'Swinging has taken on the harmonic advances of bop, if you follow me.' We did and the only time we got lost was when the literary hour began with copious comments on Shakespeare and James Joyce and Norman Mailer."[21]

Gray transferred his high regard for a well-told story into his own playing. Doug Ramsey, former KATU reporter and now jazz writer, nailed it when he said, "There is a verbal sense about his best recorded work." Musical sentences flow into coherent paragraphs that turn into whole compositions with a beginning and an end. When jazz vocalist Annie Ross first heard Wardell Gray's 1949 classic, "Twisted," it seemed to invite words. So she wrote a story that told of a trip to a psychiatrist. Her rendition became a five-star hit for Prestige Records. Later on Joni Mitchell recorded it. In the 1950s Annie Ross combined her talents with Dave Lambert and Jon Hendricks to make a vocalized rendition of "Little Pony," Gray's classic tenor solo from his days with Count Basie.

Gray wore a slim mustache on a scarecrow frame. He boasted a waistline of twenty-four inches. "Mosquito Knees" was one of his nicknames. Most knew him as the "Thin Man" or the "Greyhound" for his agility at breakneck tempos. He liked expensive clothes and was fussy about his dress.[22]

Gray's old shoe brush is the only memento drummer Tim Kennedy has of those days with the Al Killian sextet in Portland. Kennedy, in a phone interview from Harlem, talked about his days in Portland.

I ended up with the shoe brush because Wardell and Sonny and me and the bass player Shep Shepherd all lived together in a private home. Kitty's, I think it was. It was close to where we were playing. Killian had his girlfriend in Portland and Charley Fox, our piano player, had some other place to stay. We were filling up dates for Billy Eckstine, and Portland was our last stop. We stayed there quite a while because everyone loved the band so much.

We knew about the segregation in Portland, but to us Williams Avenue was Portland. One day for something different we went to the Coon Chicken Inn (now the Prime Rib) and laughed out loud at the sign outside and at the front door which was in the form of Little Black Sambo's wide-open mouth. But you know what? They had the best chicken in town. Really.

All we did all day and mostly all night was play jazz, mostly at the Savoy, right down from where we were staying. We were heavy, man. Nobody ever asked to sit in, that's for sure. 'Cause they would have felt the heat. Killian was older than the rest of us. My uncle played with him in the Basie Band. Sonny Criss wasn't even twenty but fast as hell. Charley Fox could play in any style, bop or anything, and Shep Shepherd was the rock on bass,

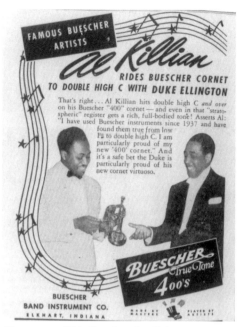

FAMOUS BUESCHER ARTISTS

Al Killian

RIDES BUESCHER CORNET TO DOUBLE HIGH C WITH DUKE ELLINGTON

That's right . . . Al Killian hits double high C *and over* on his Buescher "400" cornet — and even in that "stratospheric" register gets a rich, full-bodied tone! Asserts Al: "I have used Buescher instruments since 1937 and have found them true from low F# to double high C. I am particularly proud of my new '400' cornet." And it's a safe bet the Duke is particularly proud of his new cornet virtuoso.

BUESCHER *True Tone* 400's

BUESCHER BAND INSTRUMENT CO. ELKHART, INDIANA

(Courtesy of McClendon family)

but Wardell was way ahead of all of us. Of course, that was many years ago, but was probably the best time in my life. We had the best of everything: best music, best food, best women; all the people on the Avenue coming to see us. Yeah, it was definitely the best time of my life. When it died, Portland died for us.[23]

The Thin Man's understudy in Portland was Roy Jackson, a live wire from Indiana who came to Portland in 1939. His passion for the sea was almost as great as his love for a Wardell Gray solo. He would play saxophone for a year and then leave for months at a time as a merchant marine. It was on such a voyage that he was robbed and murdered by a desperate alcoholic, who had seen him flashing one-hundred-dollar bills around in a local bar. Warren Bracken, in whose band Jackson often played, said,

"He cared little for money. All he thought about was the saxophone and going to sea."[24] The older musicians in town called him "Little Devil" for his proficiency at such an early age. According to Dale Harris, he was in the Lionel Hampton band for a brief time in the early fifties. "But he couldn't stand success," says Harris. "He and I hung out together for a while 'cause he used to come into Madrona, where I was working, to see if there was anything new by Wardell or James Moody. He thought that if you ate enough vegetables and egg salad sandwiches, you could take anything into your body because it would balance everything out and you could stay healthy."[25] Ray Horn, jazz broadcaster, was impressed by Jackson's demeanor on the stage. "He was so smooth. He would blow licks that other tenors would wait all their life to think of, but to Jackson they were nothing special, almost throw-aways. Roy lived with his aunt for a while, right across from where Paul's Paradise used to be."[26]

For all the time that Jackson spent in Portland, you would think that there would be some local recordings. So far none have turned up. His saxophone can be heard on four tracks with Jimmy Witherspoon done in the spring of 1953 with Cleve Williams on the trombone. The best is "Fast Women, Slow Blues." He also has a few bars on "Kiss Tomorrow Goodbye" from a Percy Mayfield recording done about that same time.

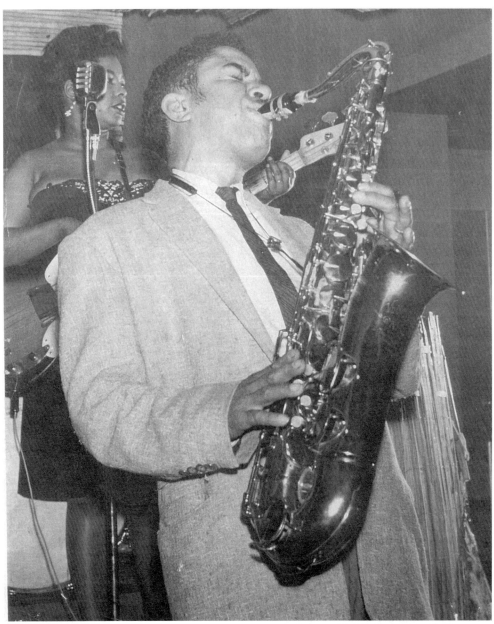

Roy Jackson with Marianne Mayfield
(courtesy of James Benton)

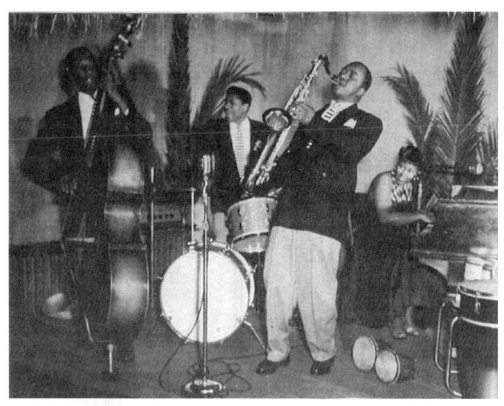

The Hamiltones, left to right: Al Johnson, bass; Johnny Hamilton, drums; Al Hickey, sax; Elise Blye, piano (courtesy of Margaret Havlicek and Phil Hunt)

Al Hickey, the tenor saxophone with the popular Hamiltones for over thirty years, fell under the influence of the Greyhound, Wardell Gray, while he was still living in Seattle and playing at the Washington Social Club. "Wardell came in one night and every tenor player in the area heard about it and rushed down to try to blow him away. After he finished giving them all a lesson, he and I stayed up the whole night talking music. I had taught myself to play by listening to Louis Jordan records and I played and studied in college. But I had a lot of questions about improvisation, such as when do you play the melody and when do you play the chords? How do you

move from chord to chord? He told me that when he practiced, he practiced that over and over again so that it would come out naturally on the job." Hickey could relate to that because he had been a basketball player in college and understood quite well that how you do in a game depends on what kind of practice you had the week before.

Hickey went to Fisk College on a basketball ride but ended up a music major. One of the reasons must have been that the great Jimmie Lunceford was enrolled there. Hickey played with the earliest edition of Lunceford's great band. But what really turned his career around was a course he took called music appreciation. "I wanted to learn more about all kinds of music so I took this course, and the instructor bawled me out in front of the class. He said I was sand-bagging. He thought that I must have been a music major by the kind of questions I was asking, looking for an easy grade. I cussed him out underneath my breath at the time, but he made me aware of my own gift, and now I wish I could thank him."

At Fisk, Hickey met trumpeter Doc Wheeler. He and Hickey led the Jive Bombers, a six-piece jump group on the order of Jack McVea. They played blues, a little bop, some burlesque. Hickey had the group for about ten years in Seattle and, like so many others, he got tired of the liquor laws in Washington. He had been coming down to Portland on weekends since 1946 but was reluctant to move because of an incident that happened after a job at McElroy's Ballroom in 1947, when he was with the Robert "Bumps" Blackwell band. "After work we were looking for something to eat. I mentioned that we could eat down the street but we soon found out that we couldn't eat downtown. Blacks couldn't even get a cup of coffee downtown or try on a suit, use the restroom, or even sit on the main floor of a theater."[27]

Because of that, Hickey didn't move to Portland until 1953, when he got a call from drummer-vocalist Johnny Hamilton, who wanted to form a quartet that included a tenor saxophone. And that was the beginning of the Hamiltones, a piano, an organ, a bass, drums, and a saxophone. They lasted for forty-two years. In the beginning they were a jump group, similar to the Jive Bombers in Seattle, a little less raucous but aimed at the dancers. It really wasn't jazz, although there was some of that too. They had the best of both worlds. They could entertain on the job and jam afterwards at the Savoy or at the Olympic Room. Hickey's appearance on the Mt. Hood Festival of Jazz poster in 1990 may have been his highest compliment.

For a short time there was mystery surrounding the death of Wardell Gray after his overdosed body was found in a vacant lot in Las Vegas. "Foul play!" some cried. There wasn't any. There is, however, a mystery about the apparent suicide of Sonny Criss. One knowledgeable critic said he shot himself in the head by accident. Another insider insists that suicide was consistent with Criss's self-destructive personality: unhappy to the core, totally paranoid, and none of it really caused by alcohol or drugs.[28] His death came just when everything was going right—he was headed for Japan and a king's welcome, where you could, and probably still can, find any of his recordings in print. He loved Japan, he loved Paris, and he had many fans in Portland. But mostly he loved his home town of Los Angeles, where he was never quite accepted. In the 1950s Los Angeles was the center for cool jazz and Criss's playing was hot. "He was a hot cat on a cool roof," said one writer.[29] Criss was a West Coast Charlie Parker in a town where orchestrated Lester Young was in vogue. Criss had an abrasive tone on the order of Earl Bostic but without the rasp. When he played at the Savoy he stood stone still and only the fast movement of his fingers could explain the barrage of thirty-second notes shooting out the barrel of his horn. Ornette Coleman called him the "Fastest Man Alive." The Black Tornado is a good way to describe him for the whirlwind way he would come in on a solo.

A Sonny Criss cult still exists among people who believe he was second only to Charlie Parker when it came to playing the Blues. Criss credits four people for his success: Teddy Edwards in Los Angeles; Hank O'Day in Memphis, Tennessee, where he was born; Charlie Parker; and his mother, Lucy Criss, who spoiled him with free rent, a closet full of name-brand suits, and a yellow convertible. One day she returned from Chicago with a copy of Charlie Parker's "Congo Blues" tucked in her suitcase. "That record popped my mind," said Criss.[30] He spent the rest of his life trying to play as much like Charlie Parker as possible. Among the first recordings Criss made were some acetates with the Al Killian sextet done at the Savoy in Portland on October 17, 1947. They first came out on an LP titled *Sonny Criss Immortal* on Xanadu, an independent record company owned by the indispensable Don Schlitten. It was Schlitten himself who rescued these precious tapes from Sonny Criss's own clothes closet, where they were buried under empty gin bottles. They are the only commercial recordings of anything ever done on Williams Avenue. Unfortunately, they have been spliced, abridged, and completely doctored. Still and all, you can get a pretty good idea of the effect that the Al Killian sextet had on the crowd that rainy night at the Savoy, as well as the blazing artistry of Criss.

Sonny Criss, Carl Thomas, and Roscoe Weathers from Seattle left a legacy of stand-out alto saxophonists in Portland, including Les Williams, Garland Graham, Earle Minor, and that great might-have-been, George Lawson. Lawson used to come in to Madrona Records looking for Cannonball Adderley records in his baseball uniform, a glove in one hand, a saxophone case in the other. He should have ended up making a record under his own name for a major label like Walter Benton did. But George Lawson "lost out to loose living habits," as broadcaster Ray Horn so delicately put it. "He was another Phil Woods. No one could touch him from about 1954 to 1958. He just wanted to play the art, man, and let the business side of it fall where it may. He'd cook his head with whatever he was taking and then he'd clean himself up. He'd make a comeback, scare the crap out of all the opposition at Paul's. Then he would disappear again."[31]

Saxophonist Dan Mason remembers that Lawson had an amazing capacity to come up to whatever level of ability he was thrown in with, as he did on those two nights at the club on NW Glisan called Delevan's in the early eighties. "Of all of the people back then, he had the most potential to really become something. Sometimes his solos would, you know, stop you and you'd wonder, now what in hell am I going to play after that? Lee Reinoehl, George, and myself came up at the same time, when everything was starting to close down, not just on the Avenue but everywhere.

Good work became scarce and George's big problem was that he had a family to support, so he had to have a day job and then he'd be forced to play with some "Louie Louie" rock group with a bad guitar player where George would have to teach him the basic chords." For a long time he was backing up strippers and bottom-of-the-ladder comedians at the Four Star Theater off Burnside. Mason says that one group he played with had stimulants everywhere, and then the leader, after a couple of numbers, would invariably jump up and run out to make a trifecta bet at the racetrack and then never come back. "I think after a while that got to George."[32] Lawson never went into a recording studio to make a jazz recording. A tape recorder, however, happened to be running at a Portland Art Museum concert in 1965. Lawson, in a dry and mellow tone recalling the late Paul Desmond, played a couple of jazz ballads to perfection, justifying all those tall tales about his unfulfilled genius.

Al Killian was like the end of the "1812 Overture"—highly explosive. In September of 1950, two days before his thirty-first birthday, he lost his temper for the last time in the hallway of Los Angeles' Silverthorn Apartments. A jealous and enraged janitor, looking to collect on a twenty-dollar debt, gunned down Killian and his girlfriend.[33]

Killian had spent a lot of time in Portland in 1947. Before that he was in town many times as a high-note specialist with Count Basie, Charlie Barnet, Lionel Hampton, and Billy Eckstine. His main job, for which he was well paid, was to put an exclamation mark on a performance. He was the finisher. Norman Granz would send him in to blow everyone away with his sky-rocketing crescendos. A good example is "Sweet Georgia Brown" at Jazz at the Philharmonic, where he is standing between Dizzy Gillespie and Charlie Parker.

Killian turned primal screaming into an art form. The saxophonist Teddy Edwards said of him, "The difference between Killian and the other stratospheric specialists is that he actually said something in that altitude. He played real melodies not just sound effects."[34] British jazz writer Alan Morgan believes that the success of many big bands depended on the pinpoint trumpet of Al Killian. One of Killian's most enthusiastic fans is jazz historian Gunther Schuller, who wrote "that the full round fat altissimo B flats on 'Eastside, Westside' represent one of the most spectacular high-note trumpet performances ever played."[35]

Killian was an imposing specimen, with wide muscular shoulders, a thick neck, and dark deep-set eyes. On the middle finger of his right hand he wore a sapphire ring that could make a lasting impression on anyone who didn't see it Killian's way.[36]

Henry Kincaid in Ross Russell's excellent novel, *The Sound,* is Al Killian's fictional counterpart. Kincaid is a high note man who specializes in breathless climaxes. Like Killian, he was a former big star of the swing era where "he was popping high notes off the ceiling but who was no match for Red Turner's bebop playing."[37] Al Killian also found bop difficult. At the Savoy, Criss remembers that Killian really wasn't capable of playing in that vein, and Portland's Warren Bracken played with Killian in the Eckstine band of '47 and knew all about his frustration. "He couldn't connect the fast notes in bop," says Bracken. "He'd get this look on his face, and man, you didn't want to cross him then. He didn't like my playing. He said I wasn't loud enough."[38]

CHAPTER 9

McClendon's—Rhythm Was His Business

Bill McClendon, one of the driving forces behind the development of Williams Avenue, bought the Savoy in 1949 and called it the Rhythm Room. McClendon says he took over the club so he could have a place to play piano. Like the composer Ernie Hood, who once said he was "born under the sign of the Octopus," McClendon had his hands into everything and a lot of it had to do with jazz. He was a civil rights activist and a publisher and jazz columnist for the *People's Observer*, a Black newspaper owned by McClendon and Charlie Garrett. The paper combined wedding and birth announcements with news about egregious acts of discrimination. There was a sports column with an accent on Black athletes and a music column on the blues and jazz in and out of the Avenue, acts that the white newspapers would not mention. The column was written by McClendon under a pseudonym. He would display the latest jazz polls by the syndicated American Negro Press. He'd list what jazz was available on the radio, and he'd review jazz recordings that would invariably end up in Slaughter's jukebox or Charlie Garrett's Madrona record shop. Sometimes he'd even put jazz legends like Portland's Phil Moore on the cover of his newspaper. In the sixties and seventies McClendon taught Black Studies at Reed College and Portland State University, and wrote a book about Black struggles from 1934 to 1994. He was an accomplished jazz pianist and for five years he owned the most talked-about jazz club in Portland.

Curious visitors from the Westside were cordially welcome. The food was good, the piano was always in tune, and the sound system maintained. There was a small dance floor, but this was mostly a listener's club, and people who talked loudly were given the stare, sometimes by Bill himself, who enjoyed sitting in with whomever happened to be playing. McClendon's own favorites were Red Garland and Gerald Wiggins. Locally he favored Henry Estelle. At the top of the list was Art Tatum, whose last appearance in Portland was in September of 1954. It was McClendon's dream to have "God" in the Rhythm Room in the next year but things didn't work out. "I got a call from his secretary saying, 'Art would love to play with you, but he is just not feeling well.' I saw Tatum working way back in the 1930s playing in a honky tonk tavern in Columbus, Ohio. A friend of mine took me who was crazy about Tatum and had all of his records. Now, if you ever met Tatum, you know he'd never forget you. So I called him personally and told him I was a nightclub owner and that McClendon was my name and he says, 'Why Bill, your voice hasn't changed at all since Columbus. Look, if I'm feeling better next year, I'll get in touch with you.' Well the year after that he died. But the whole Avenue was falling off by then anyway—urban renewal, television."[1]

Bill McClendon's quintet made some finger-poppin' pressings for Atlantic Records. Basie Day and Dale Smith joined McClendon in the rhythm section. The horns were Skeeter Evans on trumpet and Benny Freeman on saxophone. Their repertoire was up-to-the-minute 1953: Horace Silver, Art Blakey, Thelonious Monk.

One of the regulars at the Rhythm Room was the part-time house pianist, Warren Bracken. Cynosure is a good word to describe him. He was a magnetic center around whom there was a circle of young admirers and followers, similar to those around Gene Confer on the Westside. From the time he arrived as Effie Smith's pianist in 1950 until he died in 1996, Warren Bracken functioned as a small group schoolmaster whose prerequisite was the ability to play the blues with conviction, "a crazy in love but she's fallen for another guy kind of blues," says Bracken. "Sonny Criss when he wasn't trying to break the speed limit."

Bracken arrived in Portland with some big-time credentials apart from the fact that he was the last man in Portland to have heard King Oliver in person. He had recorded with Billy Eckstine and with bassist Shifty Henry. At Billy Berg's in

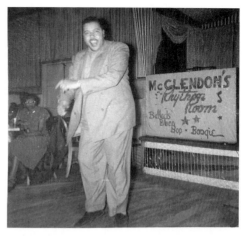

Warren Bracken at McClendon's (courtesy of McClendon family)

Hollywood, Bracken was the pianist behind Charlie Parker and Dizzy Gillespie and was part of the early edition of the Al Killian Sextet.

Almost from the start Bracken was the designated leader of the Avenue's young bopsters: from George Lawson to Thara Memory to Ron Steen in the nineties. Many of the most extolled jazz musicians came through his bands. Bracken gave a start to some when nobody else would, and he doesn't mind telling you so. "When Jim Pepper was just picking up his horn, he didn't know anything about the music. He would just take off, play, and nobody would give him a job. And it was the same with Buddy Fite. Nobody would give him a job because he was playing too much guitar. I had that problem when I came to Portland. When I first got here, I was too progressive. I had to settle down and not play so many notes, more like Erroll Garner, less like Bud Powell and Lennie Tristano. The real good player," Warren points out, "can take three notes and make you forget everything any other dude ever played if

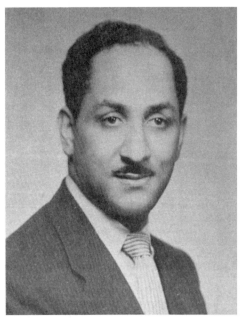

Bill McClendon (courtesy of Margaret Havlicek and Phil Hunt)

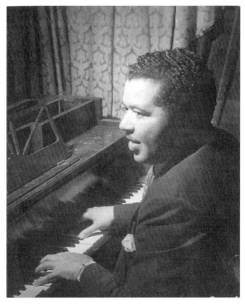

Warren Bracken (courtesy of McClendon family)

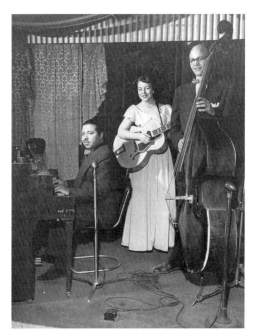

Warren Bracken Trio, left to right: Bracken, Scotty Mills, Gordon Jackson (courtesy of McClendon family)

it comes from within. Check out that Spanish dude, Tete Montoliu on 'Old Folks.' That's what I'm talking about. A lot of Black people don't feel progressive jazz. Bebop scared them away. They'll sit up and sleep on you. That's why they went for the stomping and honking Texas-style tenor saxophone and the organ because they can transfer that to the church. They can feel it more than they can progressive jazz."[2]

In the late seventies Bracken filled in for an ailing Count Basie at the Neighbors of Woodcraft. "They were having trouble finding someone so the Union called and asked if I'd like a chance," says Bracken, "and I told him I would because I knew just about everything Count Basie had ever done. I didn't even have a band book that night, so I didn't have any music, but the bass player and the great Freddie Green helped me out. Also I had a little taste in a soda bottle that I brought up and put on the piano. I thought the band was going to blow me out of my chair that night."[3]

"He did great," says Ron Steen, one of Bracken's many protégés. "He definitely knew the book. People kept coming up all night and shaking his hand and saying, 'Mr. Basie, we really enjoyed your music,' even though the emcee announced the substitution many times. When a guy like Bracken dies," says Steen, "it's a huge loss, because he covered so many styles from swing to rebop to the present day and he could swing so hard. The guy didn't know how to tell a lie on the bandstand."[4]

One of Bracken's best trios was the one he had at the Turquoise Room way out on Barbur Boulevard. Rave notices began appearing in the *Oregon Journal* and *The Oregonian* singling out Bracken's sack 'o woe vocals. In the seventies, Bracken was a big hit at Chuck's Steakhouse on SW Front Avenue with Omar Yeoman on bass and Ron Steen on drums.

"A lot of young people got their introduction to live jazz from those gigs," says Steen. "People couldn't believe this guy. He was so charismatic and he had this growly singing voice in the Armstrong tradition. Sometimes the audience down there would request his big tune, 'Who Parked the Car,' three times a night."[5]

In 1951 Bill McClendon heard Nova Polk from Spokane, Washington. He hired her and business tripled. "I don't mind telling you they came from all over, and not to see me or Warren either," says McClendon. "She was as good as she was pretty. Stan Kenton came up one night and wanted to hire her right off the stage. But she was involved with some guy."

Chuck Phillips was taking guitar lessons from her when she was living in Spokane and remembers that Jack Teagarden wanted to audition her in 1948. "She couldn't even afford to go to the audition," recalls Phillips. "She was married to her guitar teacher, Melvin Mills, who was about thirty years older than she was. All the musicians in Spokane knew about her: Joe Klose, Jimmy Rowles. She picked up the nickname Scotty from Nova Scotia. And then she became Scotty Mills. I heard later that they were not getting along

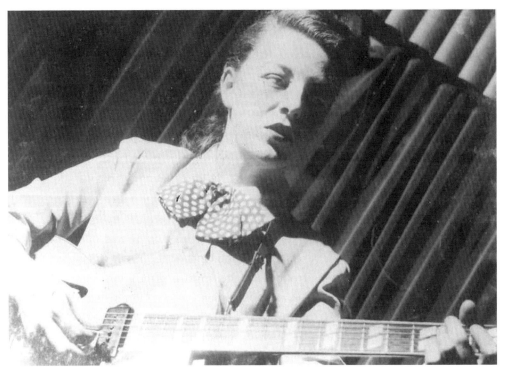

Scotty Mills at McClendon's (courtesy of McClendon family)

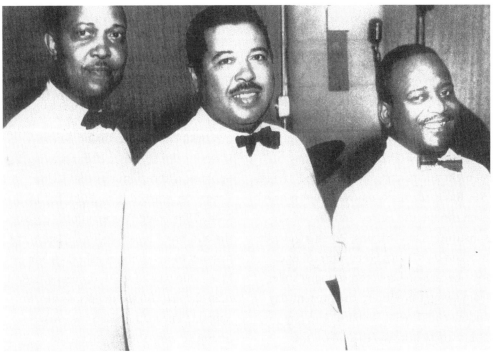

Left to right: Ed Fontaine, Warren Bracken, and Dewey Taylor (courtesy of Cleve Williams)

and that is why she moved to Portland. That must have been around 1950."[6]

She was on the front page of *Down Beat* with the inscription, "Portland's only girl guitarist plays with tremendous enthusiasm and swing." "She was fantastic," remembers Dick Bogle. "I think everybody was in love with her. At midnight on New Year's Eve in '52, she gave me a kiss on the cheek and I was still shaking about a minute later."[7]

Scotty Mills had a way of sitting when she played the guitar that made her appear matronly. The white stockings and the way she wore her hair enhanced this impression. Then with a flick of her pick she'd rip into the solo with the speed of a female Joe Pass. Her sister-in-law, Velma French, thinks the speed and the execution comes from her freaky fingers, "stubby little things with hardly any bones in them. My brother Mel could think up ideas as fast as Scotty could, but he couldn't execute like Scotty. Maybe that was one of the reasons for the divorce."[8] Scotty Mills was getting flattering reviews on the Westside of Portland accompanying Gene Confer at the Indo-China on Barbur Boulevard. Not since the arrival of Dan Faehnle, has a guitar player so flabbergasted the local fans. Then, just as suddenly as she had appeared, she vanished. Gone. Eight years later, in Spokane, her former student Chuck Phillips saw her standing on a corner downtown. "She was waiting for a bus. I think it was about 1961. I asked if she was Scotty Mills, and she said she didn't use that name anymore. She seemed spaced out. I don't even think she recognized me. She hadn't

changed much physically, still had an attractive face, a little overweight the way she always was. I suggested that for old times sake we get together and exchange a few guitar licks. She wasn't interested. 'I don't play anymore,' she said. 'Sorry, I have to catch a bus,' and she was gone."[9]

In the spring of 1952, McClendon booked an array of talent unprecedented in Portland history. Wardell Gray returned for a week with Art Farmer on trumpet and the yet-to-be-discovered Hampton Hawes on piano. Johnny Hodges came in for a week with his little jump group riding high on his "Castle Rock" recording. Then it was Tab Smith for ten days, plugging his two chart busters, "Because of You" and "You Belong to Me," Tab's melodramatic tribute to Tony Bennett and Jo Stafford.[10] This was a different Tab Smith from the one who had come to Portland playing his alto saxophone and arranging for Count Basie. But when big bands went down, Tab Smith, either unwilling or unable to play bop, went into the real estate business. Now he was back in the spotlight thanks to the early success of Earl Bostic, another alto saxophonist turned lusty balladeer.

When Bostic played the Rhythm Room that same spring he brought with him a back-up tenor saxophonist named John Coltrane, a total nobody then, a sideman with no solos at a time when Stan Getz was winning all the polls. Standing next to him and making his debut with a name band was University of Portland's Bobby Bradford. Bradford was called in at the last minute to replace Earl Bostic's ailing

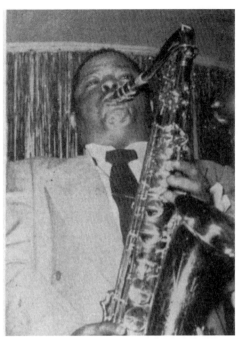

Tab Smith at the Rhythm Room (courtesy of Ted Hallock)

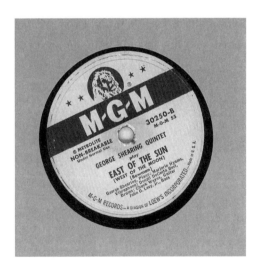

trumpeter, and as the story goes, Bostic offered him a full-time job. "Nothing doing," said Bradford, "not when there is a family to support." So rather than going away to get a name for himself, Bradford has always been content to be one of those "local cats with sharp fangs."[11]

The word spread in the spring of 1952 that the Rhythm Room was the best place for jazz and blues in the Northwest and Bill McClendon was just getting started. Bostic did very well but George Shearing and Oscar Peterson went way beyond expectations. According to the trade magazines, they were the two best jazz piano players in the world. George Shearing also had the top-ranked small group in jazz. The Shearing Quintet was the starting point for scores of Portland piano players. "East of the Sun," "Get off my Bach," and "September in the Rain" were all over the airwaves. Shearing himself had written "Lullaby of Birdland," one of the most frequently played jazz standards, a song so popular that one company issued a whole album of nothing but that tune. Piano, vibes, bass, and guitar in unison with the soft and seamless brushwork of drummer Denzil Best appealed to people who wanted to like jazz. Next to the Nat King Cole Trio, the Shearing Quintet was the most imitated group of its time and a stepping stone for some outstanding guitar and vibraphone players such as Joe Pass and Cal Tjader.

Shearing's was the first small group to bring Afro-Cuban music to a wider audience. Numbers like "Caravan" and "So This Is Cuba" brought out the wild side of this fair-skinned English

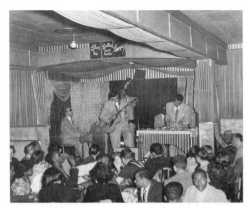

George Shearing quintet at the Rhythm Room (courtesy of McClendon family)

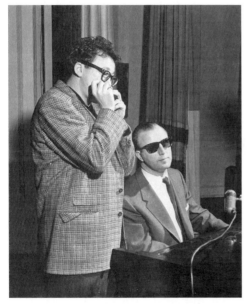

George Shearing and Toots Thielemans at the Civic Auditorium, 1954 (courtesy of Ted Hallock)

gentleman, turning him into a sort of Jerry Lee Lewis in tweeds. A head-bobbing, torso-writhing, leg-stomping personification of Ellington's "Rockin' in Rhythm." Shearing returned to the Portland Civic Auditorium two years later as part of Gene Norman's Jazz tour, sharing the spotlight with Wardell Gray and Zoot Sims.

It had been more than two years since Norman Granz had brought Oscar Peterson down from Montreal to perform with Jazz at the Philharmonic, and he was still much under the influence of Nat King Cole. When the Peterson Trio played the Rhythm Room they had the same instrumentation. They played a lot of the same Nat King Cole songs, and the guitar player, Irving Ashby, had been a member of the Nat King Cole Trio when they had performed at the Civic Auditorium in 1947 and 1948. Besides, Peterson had just come out with an album called *Oscar Plays Pretty* that could have been mistaken for one by Cole himself, and when Peterson tried to sing, it came out Nat King Cole. Ted Hallock brought this up in an interview in *Down Beat* but Peterson emphatically denied what seemed to be obvious to everyone at McClendon's. "I'm not copying Nat, he just set the right pattern for trios which happens to be just right for us."[12] Al Johnson, a bass player who was in charge of chauffeuring Peterson to the Rhythm Room each night, asked him about it one day. "He got angry with me," Johnson said. "He wouldn't speak to me for the rest of the ride over there."[13]

Peterson once said that he wanted to bring back the left hand to modern

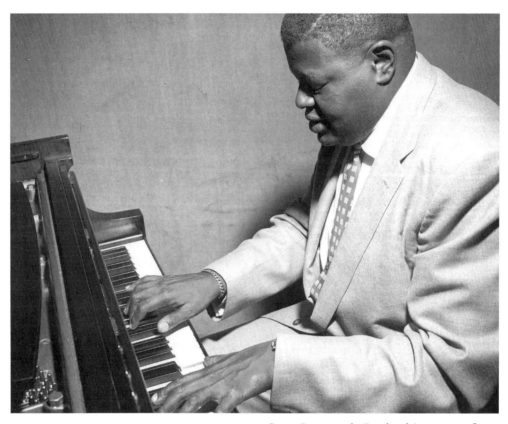

Oscar Peterson in Portland (courtesy of Ted Hallock)

piano. He wanted to show that only by developing a classical pianist's technique could a musician give full expression to his or her emotion. He says that he acquired his dazzling technique by practicing ten hours a day until his mother would come in and drag him away so he could get some sleep. Peterson stayed ten days at McClendon's with standing room only crowds. "It cost $2,500 a week," McClendon says, "which was a lot in those days. But he was worth it. They were coming from all over, from California, Idaho, Washington. We had to have two shows."[14] Ray Horn, who was there every night of the ten days, said that Peterson was an absolute show stopper with his version of "Tenderly."

"Every time he'd play it, the audience would go crazy and he would have to play it again."[15] McClendon says they had "to turn away hundreds at the door, and I began to think how big all these names were in the area of human relations, and how for the first time people in the West Hills saw that what we were doing here was valuable."[16]

Bill McClendon admits that he owes much of his success to Tom Johnson. "I met him at one of those meetings in the basement of the Golden West Hotel."[17] In 1938 a series of meetings were held regarding the development and expansion of Williams Avenue. Bonneville Dam had been completed, meaning that cheaper energy would be available for industry, meaning that more Black workers would be coming to the city, creating an even bigger market for Black entertainment. Sitting across the table from McClendon were some of the most prominent businessmen, Charlie Garrett, Mosey Adams, Oliver Smith, and at the head of the table was Tom Johnson, the wealthiest, most feared Black man of his time.

Almost a half a century has passed since the death of this imposing 220-pound, six-foot-two figure, but he still casts a spell over those survivors who worry that the ghost of Johnson will suddenly appear to snatch them away. He kept a low profile: drove a Ford, dressed in browns, and wore a western-looking Stetson hat.[18] His tastes were simple: gin, creme de menthe, young women, and everything on the menu at the old New Republic Cafe. He was the vice lord of a million-dollar welfare system whose next-to-nothing interest rates enabled many Black businessmen to prosper. He employed hundreds of Black people, many of them musicians, at a time when the defense industry in Portland was closing down and the Black people were the first to be let go. He was the liaison between City Hall and Williams Avenue, keeping track of all the incoming Black visitors. Blacks coming into the city in the forties and fifties had to check in with Tom Johnson. Heroin addicts, thieves, and suspected killers were screened. The police, like everyone else, knew that Williams was the safest place in town. No gangs, very little violence, no venereal disease because the ladies of

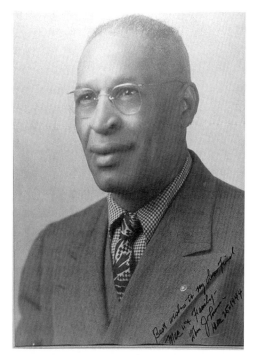

Tom Johnson (courtesy of McClendon family)

the night, always an integral part of any city's jazz history, were inspected regularly. Johnson and City Hall, via kickbacks, were making too much money to have this lucrative enclave spoiled.[19]

Born in New Orleans to parents who were freed slaves, Tom Johnson came to Portland after World War I, working as a gandy dancer for the railroad. Eventually his organizational skills and his business acumen enabled him to control a number of bootleg operations for which he was allegedly almost lynched in the twenties. In the thirties he opened Tom Johnson's Chicken Dinner Inn at NW 16th and Savier. The music was jazz. Sid Porter worked there for a while and so did McClendon.

"He liked me right away," says Bill McClendon,

from the first meeting at the Golden West. I ended up playing piano and waiting tables at the Chicken Inn, which had a small Black settlement around it. He got me that job around 1940 when my newspaper, the Peoples Observer, was having a rough time. I couldn't find work and he knew I had a big family. Later I ran booze for him during the war when booze was rationed. Tom had to have it brought in by the porters on the railroad, which was the lifeline of Williams. Tom Johnson was not involved with narcotics, and he warned me early about spoiling myself. But he wanted me to remember that Portland had always been a rough-and-tumble city, going back to the time it was called "Shanghai Town." It was filled with scandal. And another thing, the playing field was always uneven for Blacks. In his mind vice could be a virtue. You take from the more-than-willing customers. You give a little to City Hall. You invest the rest and give some of it back to the community in loans. You employ hundreds of people and you get to play jazz all night long.[20]

Johnson was a millionaire twice, once during Prohibition, only to lose it in the Depression of the thirties. He made it back during World War II when he had the Keystone Investment Co., cattycorner from the Savoy. It had a lounge and a gambling area for dice and cards. Music was usually from a jukebox. In the basement was a six-foot-tall, eight-foot-wide safe stuffed with one-hundred-dollar bills. Every Thursday a police car could be seen parked in front of the Keystone, while two errand boys from City Hall were inside grabbing their percentage to be put into the special vault in the mayor's office. [21]

Johnson's partner at the Keystone was Walter Emanuel Green, a brilliant attorney who could and did pass for white. According to McClendon, Green was the one who convinced Tom to take some of that cash in the safe and buy some property. But since Blacks could not own property then, Emanuel Green would buy it. "So Green went about buying up low-cost property for Tom all over the city, ended up with seventy-six units. And some of them like Jackies' had a jazz menu. None of them had a license. My club was the first club to have a license. So you paid Tom a little extra on the side as a blessing so to speak. Beside the Keystone, he had a place in Vancouver that was a twenty-four-hour gambling place. The house cut every eight hours was about two thousand dollars, and that is not counting all the food and booze you're gonna sell.

"Tom Johnson was the Godfather in every sense of the word," says McClendon. "I keep an autographed picture of him on my desk. Oh, you won't find him on a list of the great Blacks of the century, not with the Unthanks, the Hilliards, or the Cannadys. But in many ways he is more important."[22]

CHAPTER 10

The Frat Hall

Down the street from the Rhythm

Room was the Frat Hall. It was founded in 1930 by various fraternal organizations whose members, like most Black males in Oregon, worked for the railroad. It was a large beige building, three floors high. On the first floor were a cafe and a pool hall where a lot of gambling took place. On the third was a women's lounge. The second floor had a large ballroom that housed more jazz and blues than any other building in recent Portland history, twenty-five years of music, sometimes twenty-four hours a day.[1] Nothing even compares to the number of acts played within those beige walls. One of the building's last names was Benny's Frat

By Popular Request
One Week Only
September 9th through 14th

JIMMY WITHERSPOON
and his orchestra
In the Club Lounge of

BENNY'S
FRAT HOUSE

1471 N. E. Williams Ct.   VErmont 0332

For Your Dining and Dancing Pleasure
This Attraction $1.50 plus tax

For Your dining and dancing pleasure
Week Days, 6-2:30—Saturdays and Sundays, 1-2:30

CAFE OPEN 24 HOURS

1412 North Williams Aveue   VErmont 0332
Favorite Short Orders—Fried Chicken to Go

VISIT OUR LOWER LEVEL CARD PLAYING
SOON

At Portland's Popular Rising Night Spot—Because it Gives you <u>More</u>

(Courtesy of Bill Hilliard and Portland Challenger*)*

Hall, for Benny Hamilton, who knew as well as anyone how to bring in top-notch talent. He invited Scotty Mills with the Jackie Collins Trio, Warren Bracken with Eddie Fontaine, and Hank Bagby, the toughest tenor around in 1948, according to Clarence Williams. "I won't lie. I envied his ass, those hand-painted ties he used to wear, the flock of women always surrounding him, and to top it all off, he sounded like Lester Young."[2]

In 1952 Benny brought in Jimmy Witherspoon, belting out his big hit "Nobody's Business If I Do." The next year he had Sonny Thompson, treating the large crowds to his extended version of "Mellow Blues."[3] The most bizarre act was the McNeely Brothers, or as their detractors called them, the McSquealy Brothers. They had matching phosphorescent saxophones that would light up every time the manager at the Frat Hall would dim the lights. As an encore Jay McNeely would march the whole band down the aisle, through the doors, and outside into the patrol wagon that was conveniently waiting to take them to jail for "disturbing the peace." Some nights everyone except the rhythm section would march outside and around the Steel Bridge. When they got back, the bass, drums, and piano would still be playing "Deacon's Hop."[4] The folks at the Frat Hall had no idea that the McNeely

Brothers would rather be playing bebop. They ran with a pack of saxophonists that included Sonny Criss, Walter Benton, and Eric Dolphy, while growing up in the Watts area of Los Angeles.

Dan Mason was more impressed with Bobby McNeely. "He could improvise," says Mason, "but he was more of a legitimate player. His forte was reading charts. Between rock and roll gigs he might substitute in Duke Ellington's band for Harry Carney or fly to Los Angeles and play some studio gig using my baritone saxophone, the one I bought for $299. It had a special low A key that was sort of unusual at that time." Mason's musical epiphany might have been the day Bobby McNeely rehearsed the Walter Bridges saxophone section at the Frat Hall. George Lawson, Jim Pepper, Les Williams, and Mason spent four hours going over just eight bars. "We thought we were pretty hot stuff," says Mason, "but we had no idea how music was supposed to sound."[5]

Jimmy Forrest arrived just in time to make the 1953 New Year's party at the Frat Hall the wildest of the year. Forrest was still killing them (not so softly) with his "Night Train." "Night Train" was a

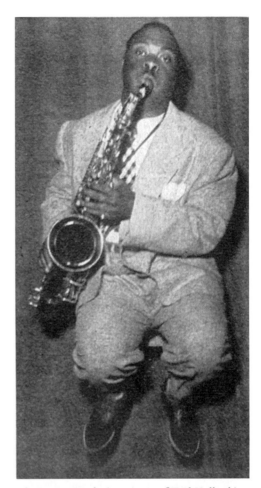

Big Jay McNeely (courtesy of Ted Hallock)

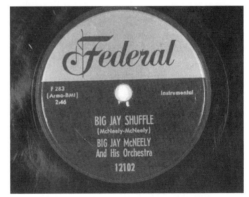

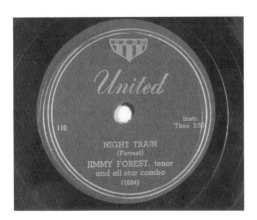

rhythm and blues version of Duke Ellington's "Happy Go Lucky Special." Forrest made a lot of money off "Night Train," but not as much as Buddy Morrow, the leader of a white cross-over big band that adapted rhythm and blues hits for a mostly all-white audience. Morrow's recordings found a fan club that ranged from teenagers to octogenarians, such as the crowd that greeted him in 1955 at Jantzen Beach. Most came to hear "One Mint Julep" and "Hey Mrs. Jones" and "Night Train," but Buddy Morrow, top heavy with jazz talent, wanted to play the jazz-flavored arrangements of Walt Stewart. Leroy Anderson, who became music department head at Clackamas Community College, was in the trombone section. The saxophone solos were by the great Dick Johnson. Danny Stiles did most of the trumpet work and on bass was the man who would revolutionize the instrument in the next decade, Scott LaFaro. After Jantzen they headed to the Frat Hall. Evidently LaFaro put on a display that had other bass players there wondering if they were playing the same instrument.

When Morrow was in Portland in 1982 for a dance date at the Hilton Hotel, he told an interviewer that he had had no idea LaFaro would be the rage of the sixties. "As a matter of fact, one time Scott was fooling around with the tempo and driving everybody in the band crazy. I walked over to him and said, 'If you play one more note on that blasted bass, I'm going to kill you.' Well, we reconciled later. That's Scott LaFaro on Walt Stewart's arrangement of 'You'd Be So

Nice To Come Home To,' from the *Golden Trombone* album we made with Mercury in the mid-fifties."[6]

Slim Gaillard, a six-foot-six fringe lunatic, spent the better part of 1943 in the army at the Fort Vancouver barracks. On weekends he was at the Frat Hall playing for the shipyard workers' dances with Jimmy Lott, one of the unknown early pioneers of trumpet in Portland. Gaillard had a goofy way of talking where everything ended in "aroony" and "ovouty," and a penchant for nonsense songs like "Flat Foot Floogie" and "Cement Mixer." That idea came to him, he confessed, while listening to a construction crew outside his studio window. "They were repairing the streets," says Slim, "and a cement mixer was going puti-puti, so I started singing 'cement mixer, puti-puti.' It became a million seller."[7] Gaillard always had a soft spot in his heart for Portland. Perhaps it's because Bob McAnulty, the popular jazz disc jockey, used Gaillard's "Laughing in Rhythm" as his theme song for awhile. It was three minutes of Gaillard breaking up in 4/4 time. Gaillard lived in Portland for a while in '72 and '73 playing bongos, guitar, and piano (palms up, mind you) at the Coliseum Travelodge and the Club 21 on NE 21st and Sandy. In 1973 he was playing to overflowing crowds at the Jazz de Opus in old town with Dave Friesen and Mel Brown on bass and drums. Ten years later Gaillard showed up at a party for radio station KKSN, guest of writer John Wendeborn. Gaillard walked into the room and looked at the executives in suits, the DJs, the sales people. He turned his head toward the bar and yelled out,

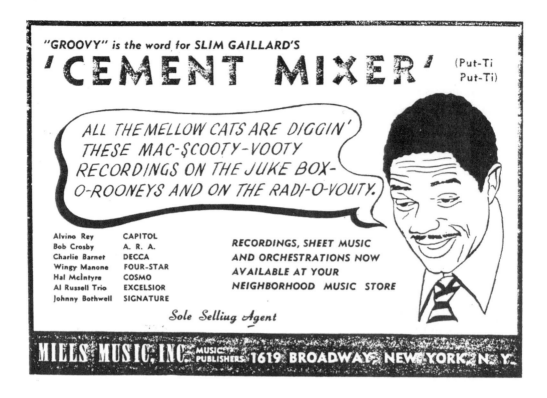

"Hey bartender-ovouty, got any bourbon-oroony?"

Fats Waller and Cab Calloway were the models for a future generation of jazz comedians, Harry "The Hipster" Gibson, Leo Watson, and, of course, Slim Gaillard. One writer called Cab Calloway the Michael Jackson of his time for "the almost overbearing presence of a man having a nervous breakdown in public." Calloway and his orchestra spent a week in Portland at the Mayfair Theater in 1935 as the back-up band for a Black vaudeville revue called Harlem Revue. It featured tap dancers and jugglers, acts on the order of what you might expect at the Dude Ranch ten years later. Seattle's *NW Enterprise* had this to say about Calloway's performance. "The dynamic king of heidy ho and his sparkling rhythm makers, which include some great jazz musicians, with his curly hair riotously

waving in front of his face, the audience in a musical pursuit of joy and ecstatic celebration, Cab was singing 'Heidy Ho' and every corner of the Mayfair Theater was filled with music. The curtains were metallic and the drummerman centerstage, and with the scintillating myriad of shiny charms and xylophone and glowing gongs, the whole stage was ablaze with light."[8] The musicians mentioned above were Doc Cheatham on trumpet, Walter "Toots" Thomas on tenor saxophone, and Claude Jones, one of the important pioneers of swing trombone.[9] After midnight they could be found at the Frat Hall in friendly skirmishes with local talent.

1935 was also the year that Eli Rice came to town. He had a well-disciplined territory band out of Milwaukee, Wisconsin, under the spell of Bix Beiderbecke, the most important white

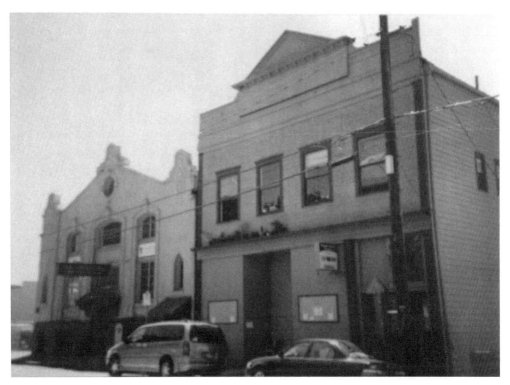

Hibernia Hall (left) and Albina Hall (right).
(Courtesy of Ron Weber)

jazz musician of the 1920s. Apart from their jam sessions at the Frat Hall, their reason for being in town was to back up the floor show at the Hibernia Hall, a building that still stands on Russell between Martin Luther King Blvd. and Williams Avenue. This was the place where the Harlem Playgirls first appeared. Their business card said, "The world's best female jazz orchestra." Tiny Davis was the star—a female Louis Armstrong who learned to play trumpet by memorizing Armstrong's *Hot Five* recordings.[10] Next door was the Albina Hall, hangout for the pianist Palmer Johnson, a Fats Waller disciple who had quite an effect on the younger piano players in Portland, two of whom were Julian Henson and Phil Moore.

Phil Moore succeeded Palmer Johnson in Louis Richardson's Rinky Dink Orchestra. Richardson, who also had a band called the Playmates, worked the Frat Hall frequently, and sometimes for Friends of the Soviet Union at the Swiss Hall on SW Third and Jefferson, or for an anti-lynching conference at the Italian Federation Hall on SW Fourth and Madison, where they were booked as "a red hot Negro group."

The prodigious technique of Meade Lux Lewis and Art Tatum convinced Phil Moore to become an arranger, while inventing, along with Milt Buckner, the block chord piano style, later popularized by George Shearing and Dave Brubeck. In 1936 Moore left Portland to attend the University of Washington and after that

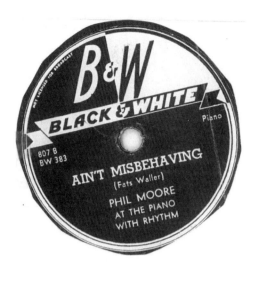

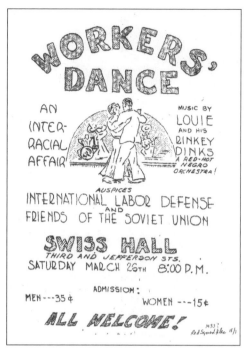

(Courtesy of Michael Munk)

the Cornish Institute of Music in Seattle. By 1938, he was arranging for Les Hite and Eli Rice. Then around 1939 he left for Hollywood where he composed, arranged, and conducted for MGM, including fifty pictures to his credit, among them *Cabin in the Sky* and *A Day at the Races.* Add to that hundreds of radio and TV programs later on. His credits are staggering.

In 1942 Moore was the arranger for Bob Crosby. In 1944, he and his quintet broke the color line at the Copacabana by being the first ever integrated small group to play at this very ritzy place. Moore was getting good press.

His good looks, celebrity, and cool demeanor, reminiscent of Duke Ellington, made him a perfect cover guy for *Ebony* and the benefactor of many endorsements, including RC Cola. Of the couple of hundred songs he wrote, none ever reached the popularity of "Shoo Shoo Baby." Celebrity vocalist Lena Horne came to a rehearsal one day in a despondent mood and Moore accidentally said, "Oh shoo shoo baby, we got a recording to do." He sat down at the piano and out came a catchy tune, a huge hit that was part of every band's repertoire during the 1940s.

The late forties was Moore's "jazzical period" as he calls it, mixing symphonic music with jazz. The owners of the Discovery label let him do just about anything he wanted to do, which was to show off some of the great talent in Hollywood who were lost in the studios, including Lucky Thompson, Gerald Wiggins, and mostly Murray McEachern, who had been in Portland with Glen Gray. One of Moore's favorite compositions is

"Misty Moon Blues" and features the trombone of McEachern, in a playful variation on Duke Ellington, Claude Debussy, and George Gershwin.

Phil Moore had five careers: arranger, composer, piano player, orchestra leader, and his final career, as vocal coach, a specialty he was number one at. "The Svengali of vocal teachers," Leonard Feather called him. Every actress who needed to learn how to sing sought him out: Jane Russell, Marilyn Monroe, Ava Gardner. Even established singers came to him, like Frank Sinatra, for instance, during his comeback in the fifties.[11] A rare LP done years ago with the equally talented Don Elliot is the consummate Phil Moore. Unfortunately it never made the transfer to CD.

Don Anderson was a conservatory-trained piano player who, unlike Phil Moore, lived in Portland most of his life and certainly deserves to be among the important figures in the early days of Portland jazz. Only Eddie Wied can compete in the Cal Ripken category for longevity among piano players in Portland. For fifty-five years, from 1925 until he died in 1981, Don Anderson played in every piano room in Portland, it seemed. Only a handful of the thousands of people who sat around the piano bar at the Embers in the 1970s had any idea who they were listening to. Contrary to his obituary he was not a modernist; some would say he was not even a jazz player. His style teetered between the classics and a kind of Erroll Garner cocktail approach not unlike that of Don Shirley. He specialized in jazz-flavored

renditions of Liebestraum and Gershwin's "Rhapsody in Blue" and set a standard of musicianship unprecedented in the Black community.[12]

Don Anderson had one of the first bands to play at the Frat Hall, a group made up of musicians mostly from Seattle's Garfield High School plus a drummer named Ralph Stevens. When Anderson's saxophonist left, he tried to get Joe Darensbourg, a Creole clarinetist living in Seattle who later became part of the Louis Armstrong All-Stars. Darensbourg wasn't interested but recommended one of his students, a young man named Dick Wilson. So with Darensbourg's own tenor saxophone, Wilson came to Portland to study and play with Don Anderson.[13] Wilson went on to become one of the most important saxophonists of the 1930s.

There are three events in Portland jazz history that tenor saxomaniacs would love to have seen: Wardell Gray at the Savoy in 1947, Illinois Jacquet at the Norse Hall in 1940, and young Dick Wilson playing live at the Frat Hall in 1930-31. Was it apparent then that he would go on to become one of the most sought-after soloists? Leonard Feather goes so far as to call him one of the precursors of bop because of his subtle phrasing and unique tone somewhere between Lester Young and Leon "Chu" Berry.[14] He was in Portland for about a year before returning to Seattle. He returned to Portland for a couple of weeks in 1933 with Gene Coy and his Black Aces.[15] In the mid-thirties he was in Columbus, Ohio, sitting next to the

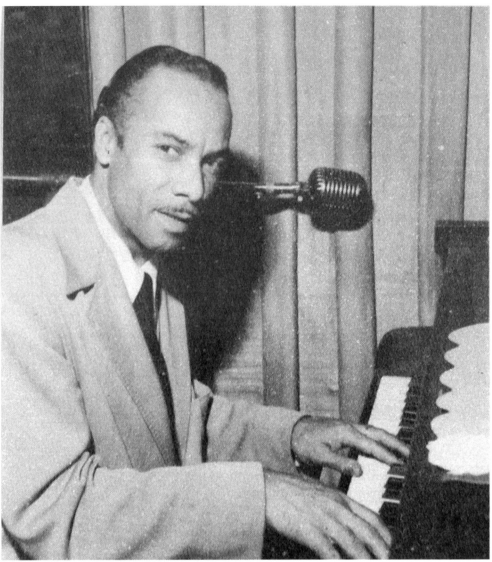

Don Anderson (courtesy of Margaret Havlicek and Phil Hunt)

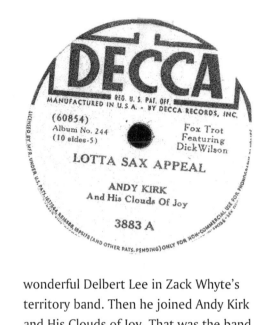

wonderful Delbert Lee in Zack Whyte's territory band. Then he joined Andy Kirk and His Clouds of Joy. That was the band he was with at McElroy's Ballroom on his final trip to Portland in early January of 1941.

At McElroy's, Kirk featured the arrangements and piano of Mary Lou Williams, a woman one talent scout called "the swingingest female alive." She loved fast tempos, screaming trumpets, and riffs that were like question and answer exchanges between the brass and the reeds. She wrote Dick Wilson's most famous solo, "Lotta Sax Appeal."

Kirk would not abide drinking on the job. "Turns fingers into sausage," he would say. Dick Wilson was the only one he ever made an exception for, because as much as he drank—and Wilson was a confirmed alcoholic—he never missed a cue or hit a clunker. It was Wilson's alcoholism, combined with syphilis, that contributed to his death in 1941 at the age of thirty, right at the top of his career. The four recordings that he made with the Mary Lou Williams septet, a small group out of the Kirk band, are

worth hearing for the quiet fire of this most influential and neglected tenor saxophonist.[16]

The all-time top attraction at the Frat Hall was Ernie Fields of Tulsa, Oklahoma. Fields led a rough-around-the-edges band, a combination of Count Basie and Andy Kirk with some spicy lyrics sprinkled in. Fields didn't have any big stars, no Dick Wilsons to brag about. What he did have was John Hammond, the most important talent scout in jazz. Hammond discovered Fields in Oklahoma, while the band was traveling around in a dilapidated bus. They were sleeping sometimes three to a bunk in flea-bag hotels on a one-way ticket to Nowheresville. Hammond was fascinated with the band and in particular with sidemen Amos Woodruff and Rene Hall. He got Fields a date in New York on Decca Records in 1939, but the recordings never went anywhere, nor did Fields as a national attraction.[17] As a territory band, however, Fields had a huge following, especially in Portland. A number of future West Coast stars passed through that band, among them tenor saxophonists Teddy Edwards and Hal Singer. The recordings Fields made in Tulsa in 1949, when he was at the height of his popularity in Portland, show a big band version of Buddy Banks. As years went by, Fields drifted more into the field of rhythm and blues and as an entertainer and backup band for vaudeville sensations like the one-legged tap dancer Frank James.

Bill McClendon called Ernie Fields' band a drop off band because instrumentalists would jump ship if they

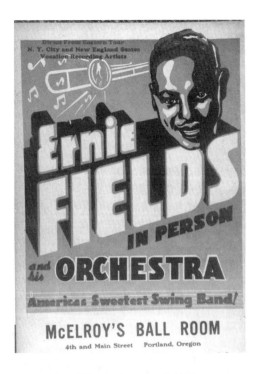

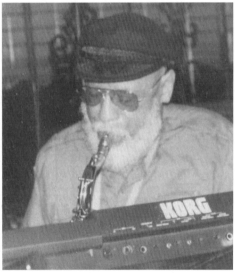

Art Chaney (courtesy of Joanne Hasbrouck)

happened to like the town they were in and no contract seemed able to hold them. McClendon says, "Sometimes they would lose so many that Fields would have to go back to Tulsa, regroup, and then start over again." That is how the popular pianist Creon Thomas arrived in Portland. Thomas was politically active too, as one of the members of Tom Johnson's development committee for the expansion of Williams Avenue in 1938.[18]

Fields's biggest gift to Portland jazz fans was Henry Estelle, a pianist with an expensive name and a talent to go with it. He and saxophonist Booker Ervin jumped ship in Portland in 1954. Ervin, who finally ended up with Charles Mingus, didn't stay long in Portland. Estelle stayed for fifteen years and then, like Scotty Mills, one night just up and left; he was last heard from hiding out in Las Vegas.

When Estelle arrived on the Avenue, it was on the downside. The Frat Hall was still going but McClendon's and other clubs were beginning to close. "He was almost Oscar Peterson," says close friend Art Chaney

well schooled, beyond Sid Porter and even Julian Henson. Braley Brown and Tom Grant's brother Mike were just a few of his admirers because he would do tunes that nobody else in town would do like "Five o'clock Whistle." When Estelle would play, his head would bob up and down, a habit he could not rid himself of, going back to his first piano teacher who would stand over him and shout, "Look at the music and not at the keyboard."

Funny, isn't it? I spent a lot of time with him, played with him at the Frat Hall and many other jobs. I even stayed with him in the same house for a while, and that is the only thing I ever learned about his childhood. You'd think in all that time a guy would open up so you could get a handle on his roots, his friends and relatives. He never did.[19]

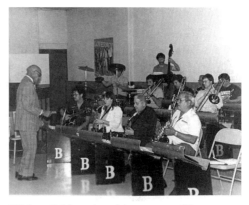

Walter Bridges band (courtesy of Joanne Hasbrouck)

The drummer and blues singer James Benton remembers that Estelle wouldn't say fifteen words a day. "I'm not saying you couldn't have a conversation, except that you'd be doing all the talking. He might show up at four in the morning looking to practice on the piano I had in my garage at that time."[20]

Only a few piano players in town had ever heard of Estelle until he played a benefit in 1966. It was for Wayne Keith, a very popular bartender who had fallen to his death in an elevator shaft in the old Park Haviland Hotel. Musicians came from all over to pay respects and to play a couple of tunes in Keith's honor. Henry Estelle's novel version of "When Sonny Gets Blue" rated an encore that night.

Like almost every other musician at the Frat Hall, Estelle was a sometime member of the Walter Bridges Big Band. Bridges came to Portland in the thirties as a journeyman trumpet player with Milt Larkin and later with Benny Moten, where Bridges says he met Count Basie. Bridges came to Portland the second time to work in the Kaiser shipyards and stayed in the city for the rest of his life. He put a band together at Kaiser composed of defense workers, some of whom had been professional musicians

before the war. Bridges' band and others like it at Kaiser played for bond rallies, USO canteen dances, ship launchings, and patriotic holidays.

In 1944, Bridges' band was a regular at the Frat Hall, playing in the manner of the popular John Kirby. It wasn't long until he got a break when trumpeter Charlie Merritt left the Shangri-La and Bridges was asked to replace him. Bridges soon took over the whole band and renamed it the Ebony Five, continuing to play in the close harmonic style of John Kirby. The band's specialty was jazzing up the classics like "Riffin' on Beethoven." Bridges claimed it was the first integrated band ever in Portland and they were playing to sold-out houses, even doing broadcast remotes "and then the Union 99 got wind of it and tried to pull us off the stage," Bridges says. " 'You know you can't play here without being in the Union,' one of them said." Bridges reminded them that there was no Black union in Portland. Then the Union reps told him he would have to join an auxiliary group in Seattle. Bridges got his dander up and exclaimed, "I don't live in Seattle! I live here. I pay taxes here, and until you let Blacks in the Musicians Union, you can't throw me off this stage."[21] Ten days later he got a card in the mail telling the Ebony Five to come down to the Union Hall and be sworn in as members.

In 1945 Bridges began a fully integrated community workshop band, a learning academy and hangout for the talented and not-so-talented jazz musicians. It lasted forty years. Depending on who showed up, the performance level varied from slightly out of tune one week to ready to record the next. Bridges was like a football coach with a constantly shifting lineup of all-stars and rookies. "It had its moments," says Warren Bracken. "It was the jazz players' night out to find out what gigs were available and just to hang out. You never got any money but then we didn't have to worry about dancers either or requests to play 'Alley Cat.' "[22] You'd be hard pressed to find a single jazz musician who didn't at one time play in the Bridges big band. Some of them, like trumpeter Howard Gatley and Sheldon Brooks, never left. Brooks, an ensemble player, still remembers sitting next to Doc Severinsen in the Bridges 1945-46 band. "Oh, he was very gifted but not a jazz improviser in those days. There were a number of players who could do better, Sid Porter's nephew, Bobby Bradford, Fran Shirley, and my own favorite before he became a piano player, Russ Hackett. God, he was talented and so was that gal he married, Jeannie Hackett, the singer. Severinsen was talented, but he really wasn't a jam session player."[23]

Art Chaney remembered Bridges' conviction and enthusiasm.

He'd chew you out like a good teacher should if he thought you weren't doing your best. If you have your horn you were supposed to be a musician, which is the Lord's highest calling. Now if you don't want to play your best and do what you are supposed to do, put the goddamn thing down and stop bullshitting people. He'd be like a storm trooper in his methods for getting a band together and he'd come right over to your house in the middle of the night, drive up to the driveway, knock on your door, and tell you to get your horn 'cause they're short a saxophone at the hall and the guys are waiting for ya. If you tried to hesitate or get out of it, he'd go into "Hey, we're a man short. Are you going to mess it up for everyone else?"

Bridges was old school, man, being part of a big band was his biggest high, like mountain climbing for some people, I guess. When I think of the musicians who passed through that band, the saxophonists alone: Sherman Thomas, Dick Knight, Kenny Hing, a skinny kid named Jim Pepper. And one more, George Lawson, whose creative improvisations made him the most likely to succeed.[24]

The Victor Borge of the band was Keith "The Jackal" Klein. Even in a field crowded with eccentrics, Klein stood out as a gangly, bucktoothed, outrageously funny pianist with a big talent and a tendency to go off the deep end, a condition he said might be attributed to having roomed with all-American

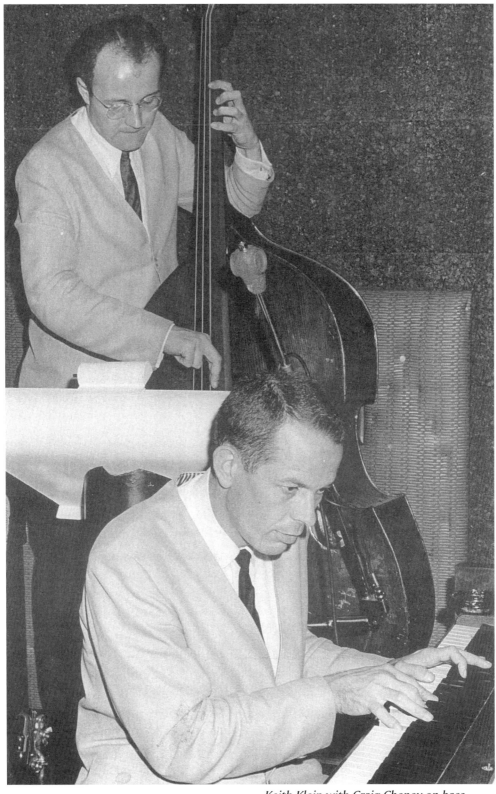

*Keith Klein with Craig Cheney on bass
(courtesy of Carl Smith)*

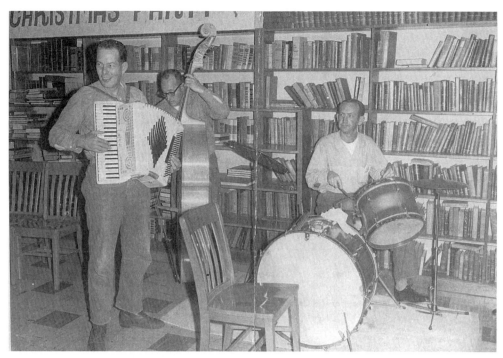

Keith Klein (on accordion) at a Christmas party at Dammasch State Hospital (courtesy of Carl Smith)

halfback Vic Janowitz at Ohio State. While an inmate at the old Dammasch State Hospital, Klein played an accordion in the band and was a weekly telephone guest on Ernie Hood's KBOO radio program, a segment Klein would call "Dammasch After Dark."[25] "You just break up watching him," says Art Chaney, "hair all messed up, suit too small, lighted cigarettes in both hands."[26]

For a little while Klein lived in "Sweet Baby James" Benton's garage. Benton had it made into a nightclub with two pianos and a couple dozen seats from an abandoned movie house. He plastered the walls with album covers, soundproofed it, carpeted it, even had a stage. It became a testing ground for jazz beginners where they could get their start on their way up to Paul's Paradise or

the Chicken Coop. "Klein was way out there," says Benton. "He hung out with this bass player from the Portland Symphony named Wayne Hearn. What a pair they were. Hearn used to wear a Confederate jacket and cap."

One of the last sightings of Klein was at Delta Park playing a benefit for multiple sclerosis in August of 1983. He was part of an opening act at an all-day event. The turnout was pathetically slim. It was noon. It was hot and there was a noisy baseball game less than seventy-five yards away. Klein, looking like he just stepped out of a tornado, yelled into the microphone, "Hey, this is for you guys running around the bases," and began to play "Take Me Out to the Ballgame" and then he went into a tribute to Harry "The Hipster" Gibson,

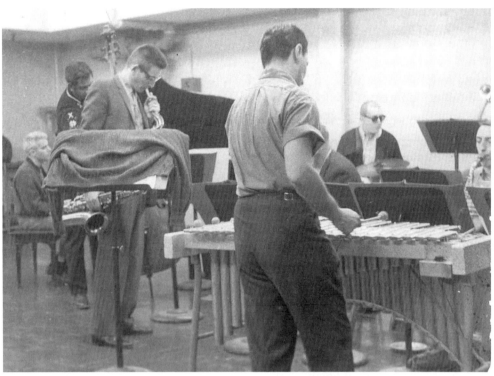

Bill Hood with Terry Gibbs (courtesy of Joanne Hasbrouck)

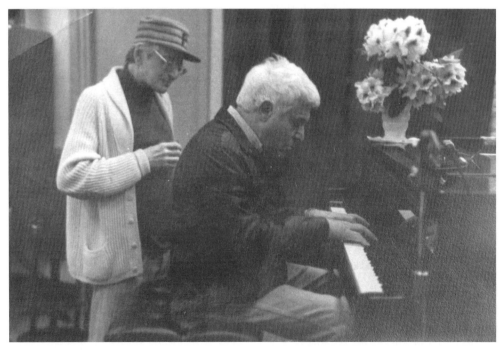

Bill Hood and Lou Levy at Otter Crest (courtesy of Joanne Hasbrouck)

"Stop Dancin' Up There," and ended with Monk's "Well You Needn't." There was a clap or two. Klein smiled, got up, walked off the stage and into the afternoon.[27]

Next to Doc Severinsen, Bill Hood was the second most successful graduate from the Bridges Institute of Big Band Learning. His highest compliment can be found in a book by Rex Stewart called *Jazz Masters of the Thirties*. Stewart was a standout cornetist with Duke Ellington and in the book he's talking about the great baritone saxophones in jazz: Ernie Caceres, Harry Carney, Pepper Adams, Gerry Mulligan. And then he says, "Another fellow who moves me is Bill Hood, who makes his home in L.A. and can be heard on television subbing on the *Johnny Carson Tonight Show*." Leonard Feather called him "the unheralded modern giant of the baritone saxophone."

If Hood's credits were ever accurately documented, they might rival the prolific Phil Moore. Hood was with the exciting Terry Gibbs Big Band and also with Shorty Rogers, with whom he made a number of records. He was musical director for the Della Reese and Kay Starr television shows. Unlike Sonny Criss, Hood was no one-horn wonder. He played all the woodwinds well, making him first call in the Hollywood studios. His bass saxophone can be heard in a movie called *Fortune 75*, his flute on Nancy Wilson's *Broadway My Way*, his bass clarinet on a Shorty Rogers Warner Brothers album called *Dimensions in Sound*.

Growing up in Portland, he was primarily a clarinetist and a tenor saxophonist, starting in high school with the Sid Rosen band, and then playing with Woody Hite and Freddie Keller at Jantzen Beach and with Bobby Baker's band at Oaks Park, where Hood wrote his first arrangements. He played with the Wayne Strohecker band at the Uptown Ballroom and frequently with Walter Bridges at the Frat Hall.[28]

Bill Hood left for Hollywood early to join Freddie Slack's band (their Cow Cow Boogie was Capitol Records' first big hit). He was in the front row still playing tenor when the band played a one-nighter at Jantzen Beach in 1950. Shortly after that, Hood began to concentrate on the dark and penetrating sound of the baritone sax. Bob Gordon, Jack Nimitz, and Bill Hood are the three baritone saxophonists associated with the school located in Los Angeles called West Coast Jazz. In 1964 Hood and Nimitz led a group with drummer Nick Ceroli and pianist Jack Wilson that got the attention of *Down Beat* magazine.[29] They never made a commercial album, but a private recording of this house-busting unit exists in the vast library of Hood's brother Ernie.

The best of Bill Hood can be heard on a Discovery CD called *Moanin'*. In the tiny area of unforgettable baritone ballads, Bill's solo on "Warm Valley" belongs on the top shelf aside Serge Chaloff's "Body and Soul" and Harry Carney's "Sophisticated Lady."

Ernie Hood was even more talented than his brother. At sixteen he was sneaking out the bedroom window of his expensive Eastmorland home heading for the Frat Hall. He was looking for Pate

Cerci, an electric guitar player with a two-bit amplifier that produced "soft earthy chords," Ernie recalls. "I loved to watch his fingers run those mellow retrogressions." Another mentor for young Ernie was Hank Fullalov, saxophone player.

At Lincoln High School, Ernie Hood was playing with Sid Rosen and his mates at the Old Battleship Oregon. He had been studying flamenco guitar with Miss Coy. "She hated jazz," says Hood. So did his parents. According to a close friend, a fist fight allegedly broke out in the Hood household over the matter. They would have deplored Bill and Ernie's association with Black people in the Coliseum area.

Ernie Hood's first brush with jazz was hearing a Django Reinhardt recording of "Dinah" on the radio. "My friends thought Django was hillbilly music because of the violin and guitar," says Hood. "I bought a box of brittle Django 78s and carried them on tour in 1945 and in the service. Then when Monte Ballou showed me the suspended chords on Duke Ellington's 'Caravan,' I felt liberated. After that bit of instruction no teacher could tap her pencil at me anymore. I'd been to Paree."[30]

So Ernie Hood dropped out of school and became a full-time musician. He got two dollars a night for playing high school proms, Greek dances, and bar mitzvahs. When he played for a Russian New Year's party in the old Russian village on 130th and SE Stark, his entire eight-piece band wore nothing but pajama tops and a Cossack hat. In North Bonneville they were paid off in apples when only four people showed up for a

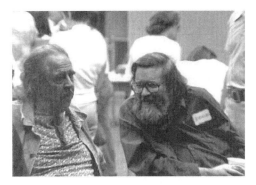

Ernie Hood (right) with Monte Ballou (courtesy of Joanne Hasbrouck)

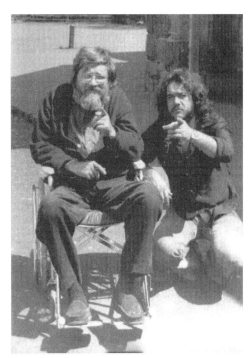

Ernie Hood with percussionist Airto (courtesy of Joanne Hasbrouck)

local dance. At the Montevilla in Seaside, Ed Beach, Swede Meredith, and the Hood brothers were thrown in jail for "looking strange" in their zoot suits and long hair. Competition on the coast came from Gene Shaw and his fourteen-piece band out of Rockaway. Shaw and the boys would travel in a broken-down hearse with a sign in the window saying "call 2 5 0 and away you go. Don't let jazz die."[31]

The radio continued to be the main source for Hood's new ideas. He heard the open fifths on Muggsy Spanier's "Black and Blue" and Oscar Moore with the Nat King Cole Trio. He went absolutely wild and wore the grooves gray listening to Charlie Barnet's guitar player Bus Etri playing "Wandering Blues." More than anything, though, hearing Stan Kenton at Jantzen Beach in 1941 was, until the day he died, Ernie Hood's most thrilling musical experience.

Ernie was in the service for part of 1943. When he got out, Ed Beach, Al Wied, and Ernie formed a trio shamelessly plagiarizing the early Nat King Cole Decca recordings. They had a following at Jack and Jill's way out on SE Stark Street, past the city limits, and at the Tropics Club on SW 10th and Yamhill before taking the group on the road.

When Charlie Barnet's band showed up to play at Jantzen Beach, he was looking for a guitar player. Frances Shirley of the fabulous Shirley sisters was playing trumpet with Barnet in July of 1945. Remembering how well Ernie Hood had played at the Coop and on those late-night jam sessions on Ted Hallock's radio show, she recommended him to Barnet. Hood joined the band at Jantzen

Beach in early July of 1945 and stayed for five months. "I was hired right off the bandstand," says Hood. "I just came to Jantzen Beach to see my old friend Fran Shirley and suddenly I'm packing my bags. It was my first contact with the big time and the most romantic time of my life, playing in the theaters and dance halls and riding around in the bus with that gang of jokesters and all that talent. We'd open up with 'Back in Your Own Backyard' and go into 'Harlem Airshaft,' and Killian's trumpet would pin the

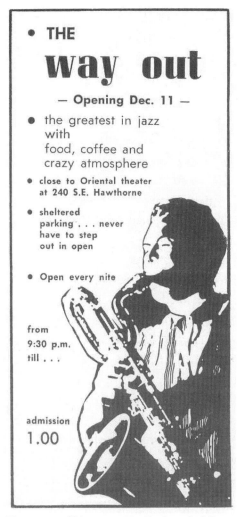

(Courtesy of Margaret Havlicek and Phil Hunt)

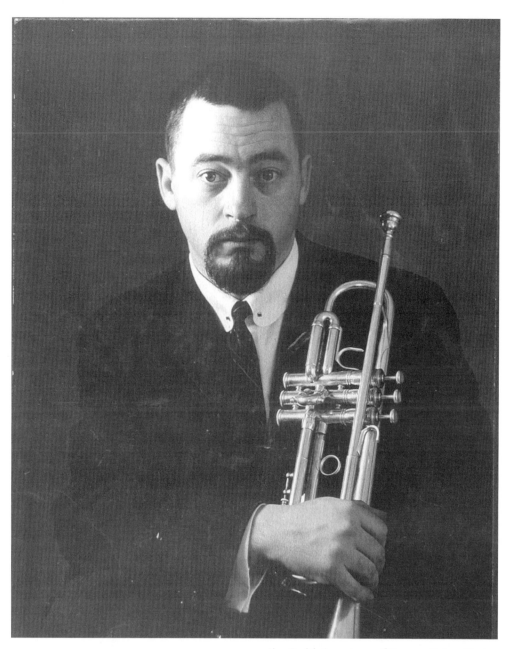

Jim Smith (courtesy of George Reinmiller)

audience to the back of their chairs. Al Haig was on the band and he had just finished making those records with Charlie Parker and Dizzy Gillespie."[32]

After that Hood joined Lucky Thompson's Seven in Hollywood, an association that would culminate in Thompson's appearance as part of the Earl Horn Band in Portland in 1946. Ernie Hood's last guitar recording was on a 78 rpm of the Stan Kenton-inspired Tom Talbot Orchestra. You can hear him loud and clear on the last chorus of "Down in Chihuahua." A few weeks after that, Hood contracted polio, which put him in the hospital and eventually into a wheelchair for the rest of his life. Not to be denied, he returned to Portland and began studying arranging and composing with Dent Mowry and Milt Kleeb. He became a first-rate composer and arranger, good enough to be mentioned in the third edition of Leonard Feather's *Encyclopedia of Jazz* along with his brother, Bill Hood.[33] In 1964 he produced a record date in Los Angeles that resulted in a privately issued ten-inch LP featuring Portland favorite, Terry Spencer, and a group of Los Angeles' best musicians, Jack Sheldon, Bud Shank, and Shelly Manne.

One of the most satisfying adventures in the life of Ernie Hood was as part owner and co-leader of an orchestra at the Way Out. The Way Out was a Bohemian coffee house right off the pages of Jack Kerouac's *Subterraneans*. It was located under the east end of the Hawthorne Bridge in a building formerly owned by racketeer Jim Elkins. Prostitutes were in the rooms upstairs.

For that reason the Way Out could never get a liquor license. "I wanted to get involved so I could get my compositions played," says Hood. "I was having a hard time getting anything heard." So Hood, Jim Smith, and George Reinmiller formed a tentet. Sometimes they would split into two quintets. Hood called them the "stumbling mumble bums." They were anything but that. They were the cream of the crop of Portland's jazz musicians: Quen Anderson, Lee Rockey, Lee Reinoehl, Dan Mason. Uncle Pudgy Knutson was usually on bass. In keeping with the tone of the place, which seemed to be out of a John Cassavetes film, painters like Louis Bunce painted to jazz, poets read to jazz, and the music composed and arranged by Ernie Hood and Quen Anderson was advanced in the tradition of Gil Evans and Bill Russo.[34]

Apart from his musical talents, Hood was a fine graphic illustrator, a founder of Portland's community radio station KBOO, an authority on popular music and in particular dance bands in the state of Oregon. He won awards from the Oregon Historical Society and was a noted radio broadcaster besides being a candidate for living one of the most productive lives of the last half of the twentieth century.

CHAPTER 11

DeLisa's and the Medley

South of the Frat Hall and across the Steel Bridge on the corner of NW Glisan and 4th was a nightclub with a variety of names. It was the Elite for a while, then the Shasta. It was the Ozark, the Shang-Ri-La. DeLisa's is the name most people remember. Technically it was on the west side of the river. In spirit and venue, it was an extension of the Avenue. Steve Wright owned the building for a time, and Fred Baker managed it, bringing in Big Jay McNeely and other names you might have expected to see at the Frat Hall.[1]

They were lined up all the way to where the Greyhound Bus Station is now to see Johnny Otis and Little Esther. Otis was an odd duck. He was a white drummer who wanted to be Black. So he went along living as if he were. His wife, his friends, and most of his musical influences were Black. In Portland he stayed either at Kitty's or the Medley and ate Texas cuisine. Otis learned to play drums by working through a Gene Krupa exercise book. In the forties he was the leader of a swing band with a hit recording of "Harlem Nocturne." By the time he got to Portland, he'd gone mostly into rhythm and blues, showcasing a double-barreled dynamite duo named Little Esther and Mel Walker.[2] Their conversational call-and-

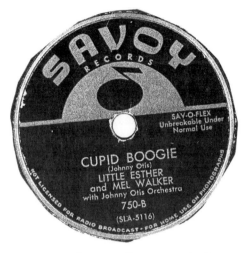

response style was a forerunner to the Dinah Washington and Brook Benton recordings of the 1960s.

Dick Bogle, the former city commissioner, now jazz writer and disc jockey, has seen a lot of jazz acts and has reviewed a lot of jazz records in more than fifty years on the Portland scene. Still, that night at DeLisa's stands out over all the others, as he recalled in one of his articles.

Cigarette smoke and hot lights were the official greeters at the Club DeLisa's. That is where I heard the Johnny Otis Band for the first time in 1952. I was a little over twenty years old and went into the club with an older and very hip guy by the name of Jasper Grant. His cousin, Laird Bell, was Johnny Otis's drummer. The room was hot and it sizzled with energy that was transmitted back and forth between the band and the dancers on the floor. The beat on most of the tunes that Otis played was an incessant shuffle played at various tempos and driven along by the drummer. It was so hot on the bandstand, and the combination of stage lights and all that exertion caused the men to loosen their ties and unbutton their shirts and still the perspiration dripped. Each of the seven or eight band members had a mason jar on the floor beneath their chairs. From time to time the sidemen would take a sip of what I believed in my innocence to be water. There were plenty of good riffs that came from these horns as well as some wailing blues. Otis was the possessor of dark, suave good looks. He began one tune on the vibes and then he'd take over the drums, and then he'd play a chorus or two before moving on and taking over the pianist's chair. Nobody was enjoying the performance more than Otis, the consummate showman. Then the star took the stage. That was his singer, Little Esther, later known as Esther Phillips, complete with her familiar and heartfelt nasal blues sound. The audience couldn't hold back their ecstatic shouts and hollers.[3]

Duke Ellington's star trumpeter, Cootie Williams, played DeLisa's with guest artist Dinah Washington, who already had a big fan club from her days with Lionel Hampton. On the strength of his giant jukebox hit "RM Blues," Roy Milton and his Solid Senders also drew large crowds to Delisa's. Milton, who called himself the grandfather of rhythm and blues, had one of the last jump bands. "One squeal shy of Louis Jordan and a beat from Lionel Hampton," said *Down Beat.*[4]

Erroll Garner played the cafe in the summer of 1951. Every piano player who wasn't working that night crammed themselves into Baker's hot and stuffy room to hear the man whose version of David Raksin's "Laura" had become one of the piano classics of the early fifties. The Elf himself appeared, a cigarette in one hand, a coffee cup in the other. His lacquered hair glistened in the spotlight as he adjusted the telephone book he liked to sit on when he played the piano. He nodded to the audience, then to the drummer and to the bass player before plunging into one of those Cecil B. DeMille introductions to a rousing rendition of "When Johnny Comes Marching Home" (a salute to our G.I.s in Korea). Next was "Penthouse Serenade" and then the one everyone had come to hear, "Laura."[5]

A cloudburst of applause followed him offstage where a *Down Beat* writer named Ted Hallock was waiting with a few questions. Hallock learned that Garner never practiced, couldn't read music, learned to play jazz from listening to records and from taking a few lessons from Dodo Marmarosa's teacher. Garner said he liked to play close to the melody because that was what the public wanted and in turn he felt he was improving the overall taste of the public. Unlike so many other leaders, he liked it when people danced to his trio. Erroll Garner's

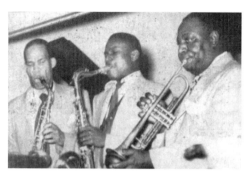

Cootie Williams and cohorts (courtesy of Ted Hallock)

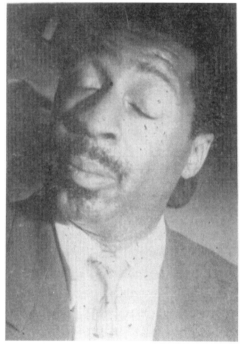

Erroll Garner relaxin' at DeLisa's (courtesy of Ted Hallock)

popularity peaked in 1957, when owning a copy of *Concert by the Sea* was the mark of the cultured coed.

Another building Steve Wright owned was the Medley Hotel on Interstate and Albina; it is no longer there. There were a few hotels for Blacks on the northwest side of the Steel Bridge between Flanders and Everett. The Medley was it on the east side. On the main floor were two bright and bubbly jukeboxes stocked with Count Basie records. To the right of the foyer was the Blue Room, a spacious lounge with wall-to-wall mirrors, fancy drapes, and a reputation for attracting female vocalists passing through town. If Erskine Hawkins happened to be at the Uptown on Burnside, it's a good bet that either Dolores Brown or Effie Smith, or Ida "Knock Me a Kiss" James would be at the Blue Room sometime after midnight sitting in with Wilbur Hobbs, the Blue Room's perennial pianist.[6] About the only item to escape the wrecking ball was a guest book showing the names of hundreds of jazz musicians, including the signatures of Dizzy Gillespie and his orchestra from the time they spent there in 1949.[7]

CHAPTER 12

The Chicken Coop: Sid's Nest

The Chicken Coop, a satellite of the Williams Avenue scene, used to be located at 24th and NE Irving, right off of Sandy. It is just a parking lot now, but then the Coop wasn't much to look at anyway. It was backed up against an apartment house whose tenants continually complained about drum solos at three in the morning. For some reason the city never closed it down. On the outside was a small neon sign above an amber paneled door. Inside were a candle-lit room with a low ceiling, a raised area for the band, lots of wrought iron, and the best chicken sandwiches in town.[1]

Dick and Jane Kirk opened the Coop in 1937. Jane Kirk was always there; not too much is known about Dick. In all that time, from 1937 until they closed in 1958, they never booked a band, never advertised, and, except for a couple of people, no one was ever paid. It was strictly for jam sessions. It might just as well have been closed during the daytime for as much business as they did. Prime time was 1 a.m. to 7 a.m., and you never knew who was going to show up: Johnny Hodges from the Ellington band one night, Don Fagerquist from Les Brown the next. Local musicians figured they hadn't passed their final exam until they tried their skills with the world-class

players at the Chicken Coop. This was no place for Dixieland or rhythm and blues; it was all swing and bop.

Eddie Wied remembers Hank Jones sitting in after a 1952 Jazz at the Philharmonic concert at the Civic Auditorium. Warren Bracken remembers sidemen from the Lionel Hampton Band coming into the Coop in 1950 after a date at Jantzen Beach. Every jazz soloist booked into this town either headed for the Avenue or the Coop when their job was over.

Only three people ever got paid for working at the Coop: Warren Black, Sid Porter, and Sleepy Williams, a hash-slinger and former dining-car waiter. Williams, with eyelids set at half-mast, was Williams Avenue's arch-patron and an authority on Black jazz played in Portland. Williams had arrived from Shreveport, Louisiana, two years before the Coop opened, at a time when there was only Charlie Garrett's Ballot Box and the Frat Hall on Williams Avenue and when most of the Blacks lived south of Broadway to the river. Williams has seen it all: Sammy Davis at the Subway Grill, Ernie Fields at the Hall, Wardell Gray at the Savoy, and his main man, Erskine Hawkins, at the Uptown. " 'Jumpin' at the Julep Joint' was his big song," says Williams, "and we used to stand around

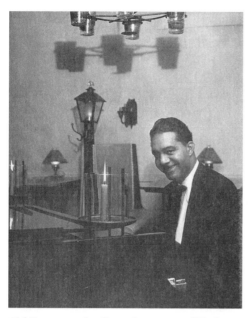

Sid Porter at the Coop (courtesy of Ted Hallock)

the bandstand and sing it right with him. 'Dynamite under every chair, we all know 'cause they put it there, jumpin' at the Julep Joint.' After it was over, Heywood Henry, the Bascomb Brothers, and other members of the band would drive to the Coop."[2]

Sid Porter was the centerpiece and main reason why the Chicken Coop is still one of the most talked-about jazz clubs in Portland history. He told an interviewer that he began working weekends at the Chicken Coop in 1937. The rest of the time he was playing at Tom Johnson's Chicken Inn on NW Savier and 16th and at the Park Avenue Club, later to be called the Cherokee, where he met Ernie and Bill Hood. Jane Kirk made him an offer he couldn't turn down, which amounted to basically running the place, being the piano player and jam-session organizer, and chief sandwich maker.

Sid Porter's mother decided he was going to play the piano when she saw the size of his hands. Hands that later could stretch practically an octave and a half. She started him right off at eight years old and Porter resisted. He'd rather be out playing with his friends than practicing. "If she hadn't made me practice, I wouldn't be playing piano today. It's that simple." Also at that time he was learning the basics of music from Burt Turner at the YWCA on Tillamook and Williams. Sid didn't even play jazz until he was fourteen. His style was mostly based on the classics. Art Tatum was supreme, but Porter identified more with Walter Gross, Herman Chittison, Erroll Garner, and Teddy Wilson, whom he confessed he imitated. What distinguished Porter from so many other piano players in Portland was that he knew every popular song in every key and all the correct chord changes. This came in handy when he wanted to discourage what he called "aggressive sitter-inners." He would call "Satin Doll" in B and they would be lost.[3]

Eddie Wied learned a few things from Sid Porter the first time he was in Portland in 1941, and Ed Beach thinks that Porter's role as a teacher is really underappreciated. "I was one of those young Turks on the piano with noise on my mind, beating up that old spinet, Sid sitting back in the kitchen with that caustic eye and elfin smile and never saying a word. Once I asked him about Art Tatum in an effort to draw him out and all Sid said was, 'Yeah, yeah, man, the best.' " The venerable Pat George, who spent the nineties playing "King

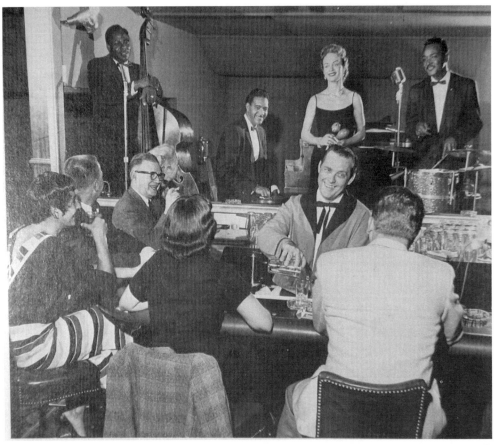

Sid Porter in his club, Sidney's (courtesy of Dick and Nola Bogle)

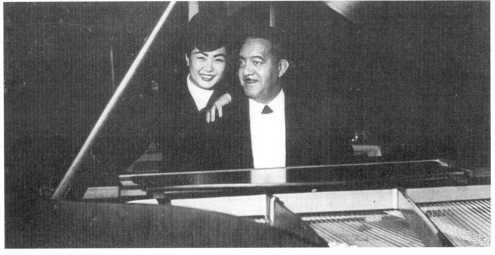

Nola and Sid Porter (courtesy of Dick and Nola Bogle)

Cole" style piano at Salishan, remembers how Porter would be making coleslaw in the kitchen and yelling out chords whenever George would get lost. Then there was Harry Gillgam running back to the Coop after his job wanting to show Porter what new voicings he had just learned. Ted Hallock remembers those amazing Chico Marx-like runs and the exclamation mark with the index finger. Herbie Hall thanks Sid Porter for showing him what chords to play and for taking him aside and telling him that if he wanted to succeed musically, he had to learn how to play in all keys. Hall took him at his word, spent months learning to become a complete piano player, and eventually became a sought-after accompanist. Currently Hall is playing a Steinway next to the escalator on the second floor at Nordstroms in the Lloyd Center. "I dig it, man," looking like Claude Thornhill, the bandleader. "No nightclub hours, no nightclub owners to worry about. I can play what I want and what I want to play is not what they apparently want to hear in clubs these days, like 'Some Other Spring.' Nice tune huh?"

The Chicken Coop closed in 1958, about the time when most of the clubs on Williams were closing. So Porter opened his own club called Sidney's at Lincoln and SW 5th. It's still there. But now it's a blues club called the Candlelight Room. His popularity boomed. Sidney's was where the Who's Who of Portland gathered. Writers, artists, politicians, people who weren't even sure what jazz was, stopped by for a nightcap. There were two things about

Porter that never changed: you never saw him without his tuxedo and he never seemed to leave the piano. The rest of his sidemen—Wayne Hearn, Harvey Garnett, Jerry Magill, Pudgy Knutson—all took breaks, but not Porter. The popular columnist for the *Oregon Journal*, Doug Baker, picked up on this and wrote a column about it. "Sid rarely left his piano and the jazz came non-stop, but he never missed anything either, not a movement. It was his club and you got the impression that nobody who ever worked for him ever stole a dime from the till because even in that darkened cave, Sid was there, working his magic at the keyboard while his infra-red lights were everywhere."[4]

Porter was suave, ultra cool, handsome—Cesar Romero. A fan said, "It was like out of that 'Peter Gunn' show from the late 1950s and early 1960s. When you walked into Sidney's, he might break into a musical quote relating to your scene, like when he spots you coming in the door, a personal thing that maybe no one knows about but you and Sid. He could turn your day around. Does that define cool or what?"

When he died in 1970, three thousand people showed up at the Hoyt Hotel to pay respects. The governor, Tom McCall, was there. He said, "Sid Porter was more than a great piano player. He was a gentleman's gentleman and an asset to the community, all six-foot-seven of him." John Wendeborn wrote, "The piano became a toy when he scooted his six-foot-seven-inch frame up to the keyboard." The editors at *The Oregonian* wrote a very warm remembrance, and

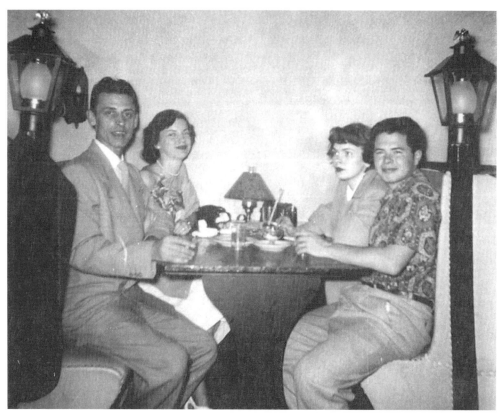

Bassist Earl Whitney, Pat George, and friends checking out Sidney Porter (courtesy of Earl Whitney)

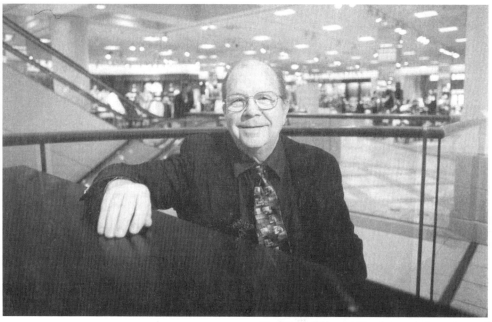

Herbie Hall live at Nordstrom's (courtesy of the author)

John Salisbury, the broadcaster, did a radio show with Porter's favorite singer and wife, Nola, now Nola Bogle. Later Nola, with the help of Ernie Hood, put out a double album of Porter's recordings. Side one contains five selections from the Chicken Coop with Harvey Garnett on drums and Omar Yeoman on bass. It's called *I Remember Sidney, Portland's Gentle Giant.* In the album's liner notes the always eloquent Ernie Hood summed up Porter's life in one word, "romance," the one he had with Portland. "He was ever attentive to her. He never left her for the glitter of big time. He didn't need to, the city loved him. Others wrote the music. Great musicians came to sit in, but Sidney made it all happen. He served up a romantic art as magnificently as a chef de cuisine. How many marriages and rip-roaring affairs trace their origin to within earshot of a highball, a chicken sandwich, and Sid's clinking piano? Indeed he was the magic ingredient of Portland's shimmering nightlife."

Maybe the most lovable and certainly one of the most unforgettable characters at the Coop and on the Avenue was Braley Brown. He has been gone over thirty years. But the mention of his name still elicits a smile from anyone who remembered him. The soul of the Chicken Coop was of course Sid Porter; Brown was one of its best-remembered spirits. His rib-cracking comments and cheer-leading proclivities made him the life of the jam session. He was an accomplished saxophonist and bassist, a member of the Portland Junior Symphony for a while. Brown was a street poet, a

coiner of expressions English teachers call inverted syntax or upside-down clichés. "Well I guess I'll turn myself in," Brown would say as he was about to exit a session, or "Never leave a turn unstoned." You asked him how he was doing and he'd say, "I'm better all over than I am in any one place." And finding himself in an unresolvable argument one day, he came out with, "How can you keep talking when I'm interrupting?"

Brown was a dead ringer for Bohemian Brew Moore, a pale, frumpled-looking saxophonist, whose playing Brown considered second only to that of Stan Getz. Brown's joyful beaming face began showing up at the Coop in 1941 as a

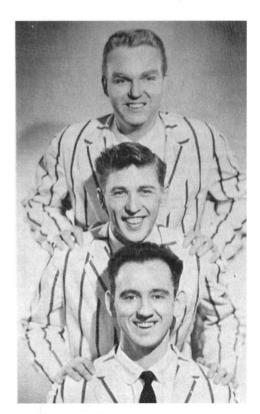

The Tri-Tones: from top: the embryonic Braley Brown, Don Watson, Al DiVito (courtesy of Margaret Havlicek and Phil Hunt)

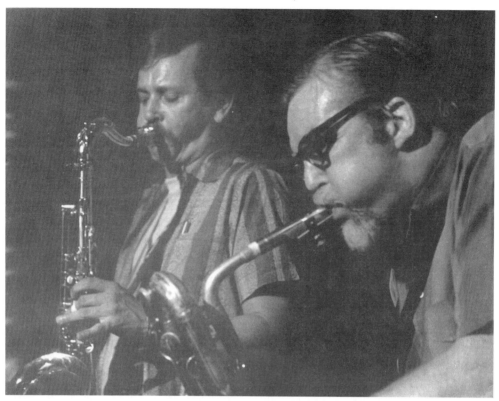

Carl Smith and Braley Brown (courtesy of Carl Smith)

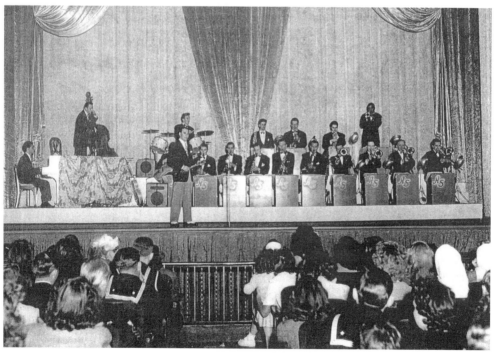

Ralph Rosenlund with Artie Shaw's band (courtesy of Ralph Rosenlund)

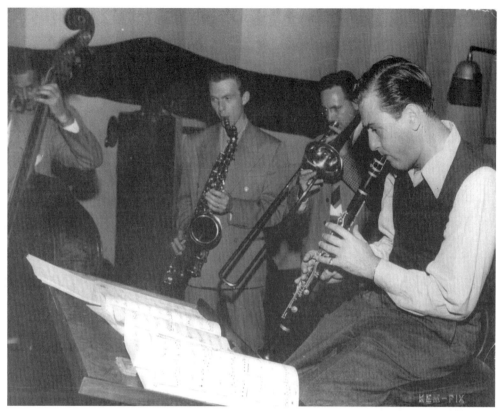

Left to right: unknown, bass; Ralph Rosenlund, tenor sax; unknown, trombone; Artie Shaw, clarinet (courtesy of Ralph Rosenlund)

sixteen-year-old would-be bass player. Porter schooled him along to where he was skilled enough to become a regular at the jam sessions. Brown had a lot of day jobs. He worked in a record store for a while. He taught music. He was a lifeguard. He spent some time teaching mentally disabled children music and poetry when they couldn't respond to language. He had a nickname for all of them, even one for his own son, Lumpy. Brown's wife said that, as a young man, he got a job as a window designer for a Roberts Brothers clothing store. Bored and feeling mischievous one day, he outfitted a couple of mannequins in the latest spring attire, then hung them by their ankles with an inscription at the bottom that read, "Spring Can Really Hang You Up the Most," Brown's favorite song. The manager fired him instantly, then tried to hire him back when the store got busy with customers wanting to meet this very creative window dresser.[5]

When the Chicken Coop closed, Braley Brown played all over the state. He was at the Turquoise Room, the Tillicum, at Ray's Helm with Leroy Vinnegar near the Lloyd Center, at the Hole in the Wall in Cannon Beach with Jim Smith, and more importantly in a series of young people's concerts at various recreation centers with his own group he called "Braley's Brown Bag." John Lawes was the drummer. The bass player, Fred Hard, had been teaching the virtues of John Milton at Reed College for eight years before deciding to become a full-time musician. On piano was one of the serious losses to San Francisco, composer Larry Dunlap.

Hundreds of people showed up for Brown's memorial at the White Eagle Club on Russell. It seemed that anyone who ever played with him was there that night, which was most of the musicians in Portland. There was a rap session and then a jam session that lasted till the following morning. Sitting on a chair in the middle of the stage was Buck, Braley Brown's baritone saxophone, a red carnation neatly attached to the lip of its bell.[6]

The man who set the pace on saxophone at the Chicken Coop in the early forties was Ralph Rosenlund. The tall, red-haired, big-toned tenor was so good, bandleader Artie Shaw hired him in 1945. In 1984 he sat down for a radio interview at Oregon Public Broadcasting and talked about that and those times at the Chicken Coop when he was engaging in friendly tenor battles with Vancouver's Dick Knight.

Knight had such beautiful tone, and very good ideas. We loved sitting in on the same sessions, exchanging ideas on songs we liked to play, anticipating each other. We really got things going. He was more into Coleman Hawkins and I favored Ben Webster. This may shock you, but I never had a lesson. I started playing at thirteen; that was in 1933 in the heart of the Depression. A door-to-door salesman from Portland Music came by selling saxophones. My sisters were musicians and my parents thought it would be a good idea for me. The salesman sat me down and wrote a number over every note in the book and said, "If it says 'three,' push the third finger down" and that was it.

I went to Grant High School, where they have always had a very good music department and I played in the band there. That's where I learned to read and transpose. I played in Johnny Callahan's band, who was going to Grant and had a high school band there. I got interested in jazz somewhere around 1936. In 1938 I was working in one of those tenor bands, or as they used to call it, a hotel band. You turned on the radio every night and they would be broadcasting remote from the St. Francis in San Francisco; they were everywhere. About that time I heard Count Basie's "Blue and Sentimental," featuring Herschel Evans. Of course everybody was playing it. I still think it's a favorite, along with an even more important record, Coleman Hawkins' "Body and Soul," which you had to play in those days. It was a requirement, a way other tenor players judged you. What impressed me more than anything, though, was when Ben Webster joined Duke Ellington in 1940 and made those recordings of "All Too Soon" and "Chelsea Bridge." In about 1941 I was playing with the Woody Hite band, a very good band, especially when Milt Kleeb was doing the arrangements. Then I was in the service for two and a

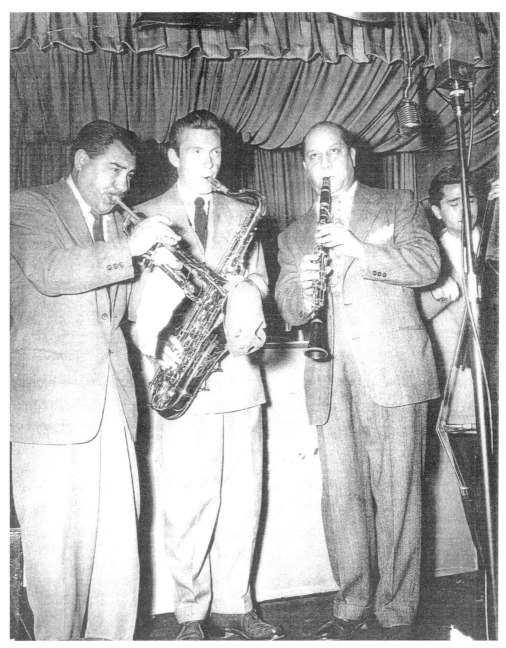

Left to right: Ernie Figureo, Ralph Rosenlund, Barney Bigard (courtesy of Ralph Rosenlund)

half years, and it was in the Air Force band out in the Portland base that I gained the kind of confidence it took to play in an orchestra like Artie Shaw's. In the service you play three or four hours a day. We were reading constantly and had an excellent group of musicians, all Portlanders. One was the excellent trumpeter Jay Dreyer. When Tommy Dorsey came to town to play at the Paramount, I was the one chosen from the Air Force base to play with him. I think there is a recording of that somewhere.

When Rosenlund got out of the service, he left for Los Angeles. He got a job with Red Nichols, the Bix Beiderbecke-influenced cornetist, and his group called the Five Pennies that were later featured in a movie starring Danny Kaye. "Now I am not a big Dixieland fan," said Rosenlund, "but Red was such a nice little guy and he had such a good band. Gene Englund from Portland was in that band. I got to play a little clarinet. He only picked the best players and we had a ball."

Rosenlund was also playing intermissions at the Hollywood Palladium on the chance that he would be heard by one of the many name bands that played at the Palladium at that time. It worked. Artie Shaw's manager came in one night, heard Rosenlund, and asked him to be at the Orpheum Theater the next day at ten o'clock. "I never met Shaw, never even saw the book. It was going to be sight reading, cold turkey. So just before the curtain opened, Shaw came over to me and said, 'You've got two solos, play 'em

at your chair, don't go to the mike.' So I got up and blew my solos and before the next show starts, Shaw comes up to me again and says, 'Do the same thing except this time go to the mike.' It was a live audition at the Orpheum Theater in front of hundreds of people. When it was over, Shaw's manager comes over and says, 'You're on. Get your things together. You are taking Herbie Stewart's place.' It was a great Shaw band: Roy Eldridge, Barney Kessel, Dodo Marmarosa." Rosenlund got about ten solos in those recordings. Two of the best are "These Foolish Things" and "Saving Myself for You," last seen on a twelve-inch LP record called *Any Old Time.*

Artie Shaw took the band into the recording studio and made fifty-two sides in a very short time. They played from eight in the morning until four in the afternoon every day under the scrutiny of Shaw, who "was an absolute perfectionist," says Rosenlund. "There was an average of five takes for every record and some of the material that Eddie Sauter brought in like 'Maid with the Flaxen Hair' took fifteen takes." Rosenlund says

I worked for Shaw for one year and I never heard him make one mistake, no squeaks, nothing; of course a guy of Shaw's caliber could probably cover it up. He was aloof, not the happiest man in the world because the music life really didn't appeal to him. I think the public bothered him. So one day Artie walks in and says he's going to hang it up. The reason he gave us was that he really wanted to make a go of his marriage with Ava Gardner at that time, who was around all the time, and by the way, really liked jazz. So that was the reason we broke up the band.

I stayed around and started playing at the Streets of Paris nightclub and the jam sessions that they had there. One night an alto saxophone player came in and I didn't know who he was, and he was standing next to me and when it was his turn to play a solo, he goes on for about seventeen choruses. I didn't understand a note he played. I wanted to know what happened to the melody. Obviously he knows his horn, but it was beyond me. Do you know who it was? It was Charlie Parker. At the Streets of Paris, I met Duke Ellington's favorite clarinetist, Barney Bigard, and I joined his small group for a year. We became fast friends and every time Bigard would come to Portland, he would stay with us. When he retired he gave me his tenor saxophone, a Conn with pearl inlays and a big bell.

Then I ended up playing with Charlie Barnet, the most relaxed swinging big band I had ever been a part of. Unlike Shaw, Barnet was not a perfectionist. If somebody hit a clunker, it didn't bother him as long as it was still swinging. The band at that time had some of the same members as when Ernie Hood was there. We were like a football team. We had a lot of laughs but when it was time to play it was like the Super Bowl, and we got up for it and were ready to go. I came home after that and started a successful business, but I was still playing a little in one of the happiest little bands around, Gene Confer on piano, Hank Wales on

bass. We played at the Indochina. We never even called tunes. Gene would just play one of those beautiful introductions and off we would go. One Sunday morning I took a whole group into the studio for a twelve-inch LP recording. That was about 1950.

As Rosenlund's insurance business grew, he finally had to quit altogether. "Nothing was ever going to compare to those days of music, blowing my horn. Nothing. In my head I'm still playing the tunes, even now. I hear Scott Hamilton or somebody and I go over the changes just as he's playing."[7]

While Ralph Rosenlund was still with Artie Shaw, he ran into an old friend from the Chicken Coop, piano player/arranger Tommy Todd, Portland's greatest export and biggest talent, some would say. Since leaving Portland for Hollywood in 1942, Todd had been spectacularly successful. First he made some trio recordings that seemed to anticipate what the immortal Lennie Tristano would be doing a year or so later. He followed that with some recordings with the Les Paul trio. In 1945 he became first piano with the MGM Orchestra at $40,000 a year, a lot of money then. Todd had been invited to a Shaw rehearsal for an arrangement he wrote. "I lost track of him since we were jamming together at the Coop," says Rosenlund. "He wrote some other things for the Shaw band as I remember. That was just before Artie Shaw decided to call it quits. What I admired about Tommy Todd was that although he had become a big part of the Hollywood scene, he never would talk

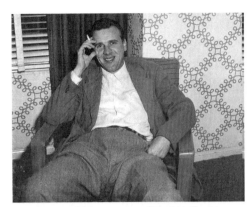

Tommy Todd (courtesy of Ted Hallock)

about it. You might be having coffee with him on a Monday," says Rosenlund, "and he could have gone to the moon over the weekend and he'd never say a word about it." Short answers were his trademark. During a radio interview, a Hollywood disc jockey asked Todd to describe his piano style. "Not easy," Todd replied, leaving ten seconds of dead air.[8]

The late Jimmy Rowles, whose playing has something in common with Tommy Todd's, remembered Todd as an invisible talent on another musical planet. "He was like Claude Raines, the actor in *The Invisible Man* movie. These days the first thing that comes out of the younger guys is the ego. You'd think you were talking to some Rembrandt or something. Todd, on the other hand, would draw a zipper and disappear. He was a terrific talent and wrote some great arrangements for Benny Goodman when I was on the band in 1947."[9]

Later in 1947, Todd played piano on a couple of Benny Goodman quartet records for Capitol. The group on which he exerted the most influence was the 1946 Bob Crosby swing to bop band. It only lasted a year and would have been completely forgotten had it not been for some radio transcriptions put out by Wally Heider on his First Time label. Almost all of the arrangements are by Todd, with Murray McEachern taking the trombone solos, Dick Cathcart on trumpet, the exuberant drumming of Ralph Collier. The tenor saxophonist was Dave Pell, who had taken the place of Don Brassfield—from Salem, Oregon—in early 1946. "We were young and full of bop," says Pell, "and we had some

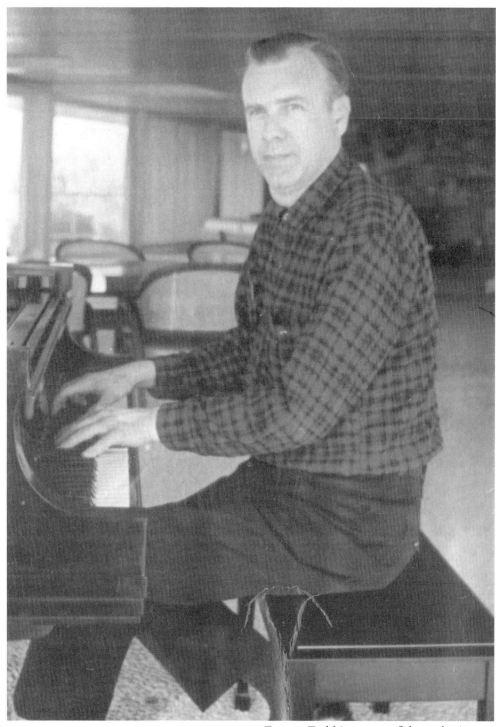

Tommy Todd (courtesy of the author)

outstanding soloists. Todd was this long, lanky introvert, a loner, who would come in like a whisper out of the night, never say a word, and drop off these swinging and very clever arrangements. They had a comedic twist to them. He'd make you laugh with his little witty parts. No one seemed to notice that he was a great piano player."[10]

Harry James noticed, according to Todd's longtime friend, Lou Mitchell. "Todd was in and out of James's band for almost thirty years. James would fire him and then rehire him again two weeks later. He is on a number of Harry James records. I stood next to James at the Santa Monica racetrack a couple of months before he died and he said that Tommy was one of the three most talented musicians he had ever met, but that he could be a big drag when he was drinking, which was just about all of the time."   Mitchell says, "It was a similar thing at MGM. We were supposed to be in our seats at ten minutes to nine. Todd would show up at one minute to nine. That used to drive the big-name conductors like Georgie Stoel and Frances Newman right up the wall. Finally they just had enough. You see, they took it as a sign of disrespect, but that was Tommy. He acted like that. He acted like he wasn't that impressed with himself or anyone else. He wouldn't walk across the street to meet the President of the United States. The only thing he cared about was Bach and Bartok. Naturally some of the big shots at MGM thought he was abnormal, which he was, because for one thing he wouldn't keep a conversation of small talk going. You

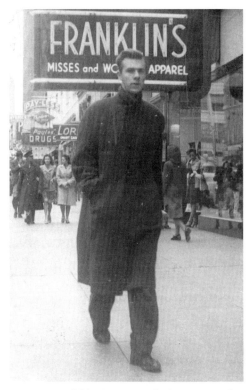

Tommy Todd in San Antonio (courtesy of the author)

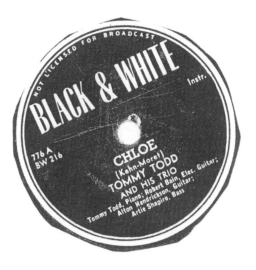

might ask him a question. He'd look at the middle of your forehead like something was growing there. Then he'd grunt and walk away. We made a lot of pictures in 1945. Some of them had Frank Sinatra in them, like *Anchors Away*. The piano in that movie, I think, is Tommy Todd."[11]

Todd's replacement at MGM was an eighteen-year-old prodigy named Andre Previn. Previn already knew about playing the classics but he had a lot to learn about popular music and jazz. According to Lou Mitchell, it was Todd who nurtured the jazz side of Andre Previn: "Now I am not saying that Todd gave Andre a regular lesson, but he would work with him and show him the difference between the classics and jazz, because Tommy could do that. The guy knew Tatum as well as Bach. I never knew him when he wasn't studying with some well-known composer like Schoenberg or Ernst Toch, who happened to be the composer in residence at the University of Southern California when Tommy was taking courses there."[12]

Todd wrote a musical exercise for a course he was taking anonymously at USC. It became the talk of the music department, prompting one faculty member to say, "We could all learn something from this student." Todd never signed his name to it. Never took credit for it, despite an attempt by the department head to find its author.

Todd made a career out of writing arrangements for which he never got credit. He enjoyed ghost writing. He got a perverse pleasure out of occasionally watching someone else take credit for his own work, recalling Howard Roark in Ayn Rand's popular novel *The Fountainhead*. The former Shaw guitar player Al Hendrickson, who is now living in Coos Bay, said that Todd could have been as famous as Hank Mancini. "He actually had that much talent. But everything had to be done his way, like the time he wrote some arrangements for Basie that were supposed to be done in the style of Billy Byers, who was writing all those pop arrangements for Basie in the 1960s. Instead Todd wrote what he thought would make the Basie band sound good, and you can tell which ones are Todd's because they don't fit with the rest of the album."

Between '45 and '47 Todd was making records all over the place. He wrote "Tomfoolery" for the Tommy Dorsey Orchestra. He had some small date recordings with Cliff Lane, Babe Russin, and Herbie Haymer. He made four incredible recordings with Raphael Mendez, who billed himself as the fastest trumpeter in the world.

The most popular recording Todd ever did was a concert with the Lionel Hampton All-stars in the summer of '47. It is known as the *Stardust* album, a Decca recording that became one of the label's most popular jazz albums. Disc jockeys continue to play it, just as Bob McAnulty and the great Sammy Taylor did when it first came out. Hampton's vibraphone steals the thunder, but Todd's piano got the attention of one *Down Beat* critic who heard "an angular sense of abstraction missing in most of the contemporary players."[13] Todd's piano solos tend to stop and go in a quirky schizophrenic manner, similar to that of Chicagoan Mel Henke, who, like Todd, drew on a number of musical styles from ragtime to Bartok to Broadway musicals.

The forming of Todd's dazzling technique began in Salem under the direction of Estelle Benner, Todd's first piano teacher. Then when the family moved to Portland, he took up with Debussy disciple, Dent Mowry. It is unclear how he got into jazz. It might have been from listening to Benny Goodman on the Nabisco radio program each night. Ernie Hood remembers seeing this tall blond guy playing piano in the Lincoln High School Auditorium who always wore a long topcoat and had a face like an "oblong Albert Einstein." A circle of young admirers would gather in Mrs. Todd's living room on the corner of SE 13th and Taylor in hopes that some of Todd's prodigious talent might rub off on them. These precocious lads, the Hood brothers, Gene Englund, Ray Spurgeon, would watch in awe as Tommy Todd, chain smoking and in a bathrobe, performed Zez Confrey's "Kittten on the Keys" behind his back. "He would sit on the floor," says Hood, "with the back of his head on the keyboard, hands over his shoulders, so that the right hand is playing the bass part and the left hand is playing the other part backwards. It's so weird because how can you turn your mind around, but then everything Todd did was backwards. Jay Dreyer and Larry Harrison, all of us just sat there in awe because Todd was a comedian as well as

a musician. There was always humor in his music, and wherever he could turn a cliché the other way, he would do it. He would go into some brilliant passage and you think you know where you are going to go and then he'd lead you to the edge of that and just before you would get there, he'd go off on a detour. Sort of like 'Roses are red, violets are blue, You think this is going to rhyme but it doesn't.' "[14]

Todd would do anything to avoid being obvious. "And he was cheap," says Ted Hallock, who played a little drums in 1939 with Todd. "He never paid for anything and you'd defer because that was the price you paid to be around him. His life was full of people who were intrigued by his put-ons, fascinated by his intelligence, and willing to be a part of his practical jokes, and I was one of them. He outgrew Portland long before he ever left. He was that far ahead of everyone else. He was so far ahead, it was ridiculous."[15]

"He couldn't care less about money," says Bill DeSousa, a bandleader from Salem who paid a visit to Todd in Hollywood in the mid-forties. DeSousa found a bowl of uncashed checks going back about two years on the dining-room table of Todd's apartment.

In the 1950s and '60s, Tommy Todd was in Las Vegas working the show bands or he was with Harry James at the Moulin Rouge. But by 1981 he had consumed so much alcohol and burned so many bridges that he was unemployable. At the end he was playing piano with a bunch of ham 'n' eggers at a last-chance tavern not far from where he lived. He died a bitter alcoholic, consumed with the notion that the reason he ended up at the bottom of the totem pole was because of a conspiracy. "We tried to organize a memorial," says Bruce McDonald, who preceded Todd in the Harry James band, "but we couldn't get enough people to come. I was the one who helped his ex-wife get rid of the piano. God, his place was a mess, a disaster area. We had to have it fumigated. Under the bed were volumes of Arthur Schopenhauer. He read a lot," said McDonald, "and I don't mean *People* magazine."[16]

Could a cranky nineteenth-century German philosopher unlock the enigmatic Tommy Todd? Come to think of it, there are some striking similarities in their regard for women, animals, and above all, music. Schopenhauer believed that the predatory nature of humans is countered by their artistic creativity, especially in the field of music.

If reputations in the field of jazz were judged simply by the number of important recordings or events one might have been a part of, then Gene Englund, a bass and tuba player, would be at the top of the list in Portland. In 1944, he was playing bass with a group that evolved into Jazz at the Philharmonic. In 1946 he was on a series of experimental recordings with Dodo Marmarosa. A few years later he was part of an album that is generally credited with ushering in a style called West Coast Jazz. In 1953 he was on one of the most highly prized albums of that year, RCA's *Cool and Crazy,* with Shorty Rogers.

Shorty Rogers with Gene on tuba were part of a nightclub scene in *Dementia, Daughter of Horror*, a bottom-of-the-dumpster flick produced by John Parker, scion to the Parker theater chain in Portland. The long jazz sequences and the introduction of Johnny Carson's foil, Ed McMahon, make this one worth watching.

While he was at Washington High School, Englund came under the spell of Tommy Todd and eventually became part of his inner circle. They apprenticed at the Coop, while performing for real money with Kenny Baker at Oaks Park and Johnny Callahan at the Uptown Ballroom. Englund left for Hollywood in 1941 and had no trouble finding work, namely with Stan Kenton, with whom he played off and on for nearly ten years. In 1944 the Kenton band had Stan Getz and Anita O'Day, a vocalist Englund would work with in the 1970s.[17]

Englund was on tuba when Stan Kenton came to Portland in February of 1950 with the controversial *Innovations in Modern Music*. There were forty-two musicians. It took two buses. There were strings, French horns, timpani, reeds, and the ear-piercing trumpet of Maynard Ferguson. The former violinist with the Portland Symphony, Carl Ottobrino, was a member of that prestigious edition. "Being with Stan Kenton was one of the most exciting times of my music life. We were trying to blend symphonic music with jazz. Sometimes the music was so complex, written by arrangers such as Franklin Marx and Johnny Richards, that we had to take the arrangements home

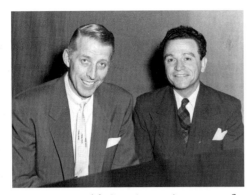

Stan Kenton with Sam Amato (courtesy of Amato family)

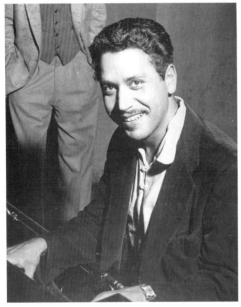

Frank Rosolino (courtesy of Ted Hallock)

and work on them individually. Stan lost everything on that venture, but I never saw a more dedicated man."[18]

Stan Kenton arrived in Portland on February 11, 1950, with huge fanfare. Not everybody liked his sound, however. Whitney Balliett of *The New Yorker* once called Kenton's music "artistry in limbo," *Time*, "dissonance."[19] A writer for *The Oregonian* compared Bill Russo's "Solitaire" to the noise made by a drunk falling over a garbage can in the back alley.[20] "Were their ears lopping over?" wondered Ted Hallock of the *Oregon Journal*.

The paper had sent Hallock to Seattle to preview the *Innovations* a couple of days before they arrived in Portland, and this is what he wrote:

At 8:30 p.m. a lanky Stan Kenton raised the curtain on a musical aggregation bound to shock, throw, and puzzle music fans for years to come. In the first beautifully shaded notes of "Artistry in Rhythm," the Stan Kenton Orchestra revealed an intellectual intent unparalleled in the history of modern music. It was the most significant collection of sounds these ears, the audience, and maybe even the musicians have ever heard. If this sounds a bit thick, it is meant to be because it is a comment in words much too inadequate to convey what happened that night.[21]

Hallock was one of the few who championed the Innovations in Modern Music experiment. In March he wrote one of the longest articles in the history of *Down Beat* with the headline "Kenton's Innovations Greatest Ever."

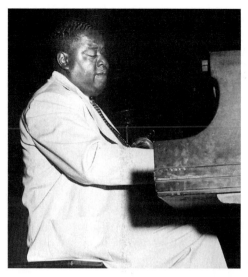

Art Tatum (courtesy of Ted Hallock)

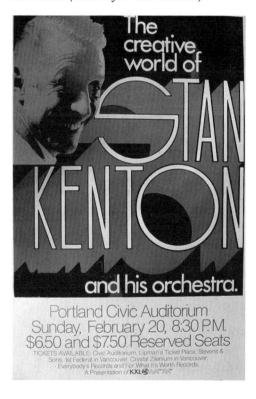

The creative world of STAN KENTON and his orchestra.

Portland Civic Auditorium
Sunday, February 20, 8:30 P.M.
$6.50 and $7.50 Reserved Seats
TICKETS AVAILABLE: Civic Auditorium, Lipman's Ticket Place, Stevens &
Sons, 1st Federal in Vancouver, Crystal Zilenium in Vancouver,
Everybody's Records and For What It's Worth Records.
A Presentation of KXL

Kenton came to Portland twice in 1954. The second time, in September, Gene Englund was on tuba again. The band was the centerpiece for a traveling jazz festival promoting poll winners of the time: Johnny Smith and his guitar, Charlie Ventura, Shorty Rogers, and the awesome Art Tatum. And then the man who most of the four thousand people that night came to see, Stan Kenton, with his new drummer, Mel Lewis, and trombone terror, Frank Rosolino.

Of all of the big bands that came to Portland, Stan Kenton's had the greatest impact. He was here dozens of times from 1941 to 1978. At least a half dozen instrumentalists, all associated with Mt. Hood Community College, played with Kenton in the 1970s: trombonist Dick Shearer; Vancouver, Washington's Terry Layne, Jeff Uusitalo, and Gary Hobbs. The current head of the music department at the college, Dave Barduhn, is a former arranger for Kenton. All of this can be traced to the happy day that Mt. Hood hired Hal Malcolm and Larry McVey, a couple of wild and crazy Kenton buffs from Central Washington. Their out-of-the-ordinary approach put Mt. Hood Community College on the jazz map with their nationally celebrated stage bands and vocal ensembles.

The jazz fever spread to Gresham and to the city council, who embarked on the first Mt. Hood Festival of Jazz in 1982. All the while Mt. Hood Community College continued to be a training camp for the Stan Kenton Orchestra in the 1970s. Gary Hobbs, a drummer, joined the band in 1976 while he was a student at Mt. Hood Community College. "The guys in the band were Stan's family and his bus was his home. He was the first one on in the morning and the last one off at night. I don't think Stan even had a home. He was a real road rat. The long bus rides are back breaking and sometimes the band arrives at a concert tired and irritable," but Hobbs says that when the old man steps in front of the band, his presence is absolutely overwhelming. "You put out 100 percent and playing drums in that band is murder on your body. It's like chopping wood nonstop for two hours. But you sweat your guts out for the guy because of the huge respect." Then Hobbs added, "Unlike a lot of other leaders, Stan really listens to your solos. He understands every instrument, especially big-band drumming. We'd discuss the form of a particular solo and different ways to keep the band swinging." And what about the many critics who say the band never swung? Hobbs said this, "That is a lot of BS. There are all kinds of swing. Critics think there is only one kind, a kind of laid-back Count Basie beat. We play more on the top of the beat, an explosive burning type of swing."[22]

Stan Kenton's favorite recording engineer was Wally Heider. For Kenton's birthday one year, he and Kenton historian Bill Haseltine had nine hundred pounds of recording equipment flown from the West Coast to Great Britain. It was Heider who commissioned the composer Bill Holman to write an electrifying jazz version of "Happy Birthday To You," much to the surprise of Kenton. It is the first track on an album called *Birthday in Britain*.[23]

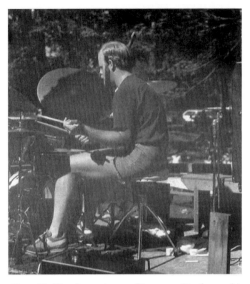

Gary Hobbs (courtesy of Joanne Hasbrouck)

Whatever the reason—the rolling saxes, the lush trombone choirs, the stratospheric trumpets, the pulverizing crescendos—Kenton fans are different. Take Bob Rude from St. Johns, for example. According to his will he had Kenton's *Contemporary Concepts* album played at half volume during his funeral service at the Little Chapel of the Chimes.

Around 1953 Jean Hoffman, a talented young lady with a mind of her own and sixteen years of classical piano, began showing up at the Coop with the idea of becoming more of a jazz player. Four years later she had an album out under her own name on Fantasy, a major label out of San Francisco, where to this day she is better known than in her hometown Portland, no doubt because she spends more time there and has gained an enthusiastic audience from her trio performances at North Beach and at Fitzgerald's in Sausalito. She would return to Portland periodically, sometimes to spell the ebullient Daryl Kaufman at the Canyon Club in West

Slope or to visit the Helm on NE Broadway. She had a long run in Portland from 1970 until '82 at the East Bank Saloon, where her bassist was David Friesen, an equally ardent nonconformist. It has been a mutually beneficial association, one that can be heard on two of her LPs: *Gonna Plant Me Some Seeds* from 1978, with guitarist John Stowell, and an album of one of their Christmas concerts called *Getting Sentimental Around Christmas* from 1983, a concert that was recorded live from the old Parchman Farm.

In the early '60s when jazzing up folk music was temporarily in vogue, Hoffman made an album for Capitol called *Folk Type Swinger*. With the help of the great Shelly Manne on drums and Howard Roberts on guitar, Hoffman sings and swings twelve of her favorite folk songs, each delivered in a whispery bedside voice with generous helpings of Bach, Mozart, and Bird.

Another Chicken Coop alum outside the mainstream of Portland jazz is the brilliant but forgotten Hal Koster, a bookish-looking pianist with tons of technique and a fertile imagination. Hal Koster is a man of few words and a few obsessions. "He used to cut the filters off his cigarettes and stick them in his ears when the band got too loud," says trumpeter Chris Tyle.[24] He was a connoisseur of fine clothes, according to bassist Tom Wakeling. "He used to come up to me and grab hold of my lapel on my shirt and he'd feel the texture with

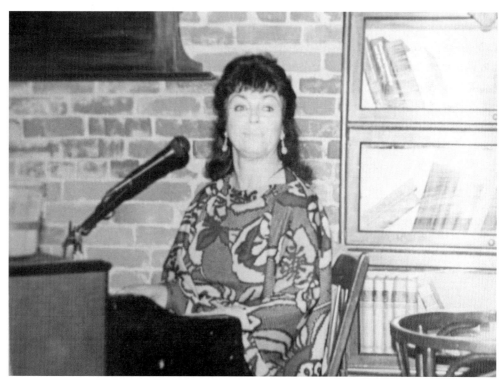

Jean Hoffman (courtesy of Joanne Hasbrouck)

his fingers while peering down at it through his glasses. Then he'd hold his head back and say in his own unique way, 'Nice shirt, man.' He was phenomenal. He could imitate any piano player, even local cats."[25]

Hal Koster made a rare concert appearance as the opening act for a benefit at the Terrace Room in 1977. "Welcome to the breakfast club," he began, noting to his audience that it was two o'clock in the afternoon, practically dawn for a guy who usually begins working after dark. He warmed up with eight minutes of "The Melody Lingers On," six minutes of an exhilarating Bossa Nova. Then he showed everyone how "My One and Only Love" should be played.[26]

The traditional side of Hal Koster is fully displayed on a couple of CDs with the very capable Jim Beatty, a New Orleans-schooled clarinetist with a knack for hiring wildly talented pianists (Henry Estelle, for instance).

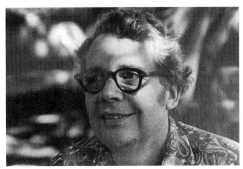

Hal Koster (courtesy of Joanne Hasbrouck)

CHAPTER 13

McElroy's Ballroom: "Portland's Home of Happy Feet"

Where the Portland Building, designed by Michael Graves, sits today is where the McElroy's Ballroom used to be, right there on the corner of SW 4th and Main. McElroy's was to many Black people in Portland what the Savoy Ballroom was to the people of Harlem—"the home of happy feet." A volunteer doorman named Harry Perlman stood outside in a torn raincoat yelling words of encouragement to the musicians and dancers as they entered the building. As far as anyone knows, Perlman never went inside.[1] The ballroom itself was on the second floor and to the left of a steep staircase. A crystal ball, like the ones in the movies, hung over a block-long polished dance floor that seemed to have springs underneath it. A shell canopy hovered over the bandstand where the greatest jazz musicians in the world played.

It was headquarters for the Lindy Hop and its many versions going all the way back to World War I and the Texas

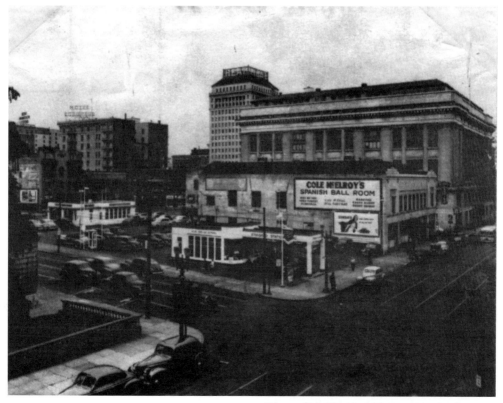

View of McElroy's with county courthouse in background (courtesy of Ron Weber)

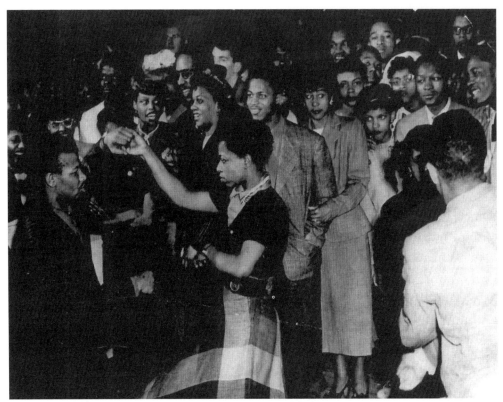

Dancing at McElroy's (courtesy of Oregon Historical Society [negative # 38668])

Tommy. Each had its own step and its own name. Some of the moves inspired instrumental arrangements like Jimmie Lunceford's "Posin'," Duke Ellington's "Truckin'," and "Peckin' " by Harry James, where couples would produce chicken-like movements with their necks and feet. Originality was everything. Dancers who copied were given the cold shoulder. When the Lindy, named after Charles Lindbergh, the famous aviator, went aerial with backflips and overhead snatches, it was known as jitterbugging or euphemistically "choreographed swing."[2] "John Jacob and a lady named Red could flat out stop the joint on 'Uptown Blues,' " says saxophonist Art Chaney. "And the fast-stepping Ellen Wood had a partner so smooth they called him Fred Astaire." Jack the Dancer could do seven choruses of the Jersey Bounce finishing with a heel-toe slide that took him the length of the floor. Even his shoes were soaked. No wonder there were so many cleaning establishments on Williams Avenue.[3]

When these exotic dances began appearing in the gymnasiums of the Portland high schools, a red alert sounded that recalled the days when mixed dancing was against the law. School principals, the Daughters of the American Revolution, and conservative ministers were saying that this kind of jazz-inspired dancing was the devil's doing. A Portland high school principal, worried that jazz dancing was not only polluting real music but corrupting the morality of teenagers, wrote this, "Go to a dance hall and watch them as they dance, their droopy mouths from which a cigarette dangles, their heavy-lidded eyes, their hard expressionless faces, striving to hide behind masks of paint and illusion."[4]

Now it was happening at Jefferson High School. A no-jitterbug policy was invoked in 1944. This caused six Black students to write a protest letter to the editor of the *People's Observer* complaining that the white couples were doing the same steps. "But the school administration only shook their head and the principal told us that they would like us to dance like the white students."[5]

The real fear was that these Black-originated dances would lead to mixed dancing, which would lead to mixed marriages. In a club downtown in 1950, a white vocalist lost her job because she danced with her former employer, a Black drummer. In 1952, when segregation in Portland was still rampant, four Black couples were turned away when Lionel Hampton was at Jantzen Beach. When Hampton heard about it, he stopped the show in the middle of his solo, walked off the stage, and threatened to take the rest of his band with him. Within minutes, the couples were admitted and the band played on.[6]

One of the fiercest fighters for civil rights in Portland was Cole "Pop" McElroy, the owner of McElroy's Ballroom. Just a few months before he died, McElroy and Norman Granz sponsored a Jazz at the Philharmonic concert in the Civic Auditorium in the name of equal rights. The usual legends

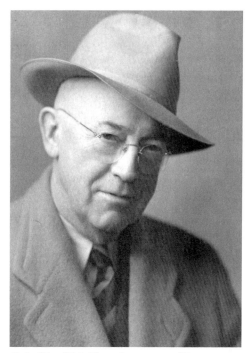

Cole "Pop" McElroy (courtesy of Ray Spurgeon)

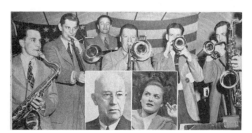

McElroy and Margaret Carroll (Havlicek), with McElroy's brass section (courtesy of Margaret Havlicek and Phil Hunt)

showed up: Buddy Rich, Roy Eldridge, Coleman Hawkins, and Flip Phillips. Later on many of them were seen jamming at the Coop and at the Savoy.[7]

Pop McElroy's funeral in July of 1947 was one of the largest in living memory. Blacks and whites in equal number lined up about half a block to pay their last respects to an old friend. The *Northwest Enterprise*, a Black newspaper out of Seattle, had this to say about the man who, against the advice of City Hall, opened up his ballroom to Black dancers in the early 1930s: "His rare understanding and sympathy for the down and outer was almost Christ-like. McElroy just loved people. He had a huge following of friends among Negro citizens who were represented among hundreds and hundreds of others who attended his last rites. Not many in life are spoken of so gently."

Hank Wales, an early explorer on jazz bass, says, "McElroy was a free thinker. He wasn't as interested in commercial success as he was in breaking down the doors of segregation. He was booking Black bands even before I got here, and I got here in 1931. I was at McElroy's the night in early 1940 when Ella Fitzgerald brought the Chick Webb band into McElroy's. She and Taft Jordan had just taken it over after Chick died. Afterwards we all went out to the Avenue, first to the Frat Hall where Bobby Stark, Sandy Williams, and Taft Jordan all sat in, and then we headed for Spicers for the best barbecued ribs in the city."[8]

If the promoters of jazz in Portland had a Hall of Fame, Cole "Pop" McElroy and Stanton Duke would be at the top of

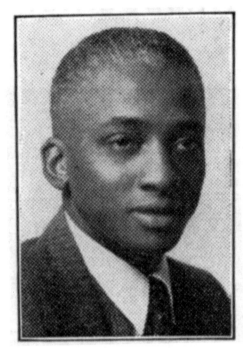

Stanton Duke (courtesy of Dick Bogle)

the list. Their relationship must have been decreed in Heaven: the cherry-cheeked big-hearted Irishman and the self-educated dining-car waiter with an orderly mind and an avid interest in elocution. If the times had been different, you could imagine Stanton Duke as a CEO somewhere.[9]

Starting in the early thirties, Stanton Duke anticipated the swing era and the growing demand for Black entertainment, particularly Black big bands. Stanton Duke was the quintessential promoter—well-dressed, well-mannered, very well-spoken, all business, and a workaholic. From his travels on the railroad, he contacted many Black band leaders who had never been to Portland. So in 1934, along with Pop McElroy, he started Bronze Attractions, bringing big bands into McElroy's and other small dance halls like

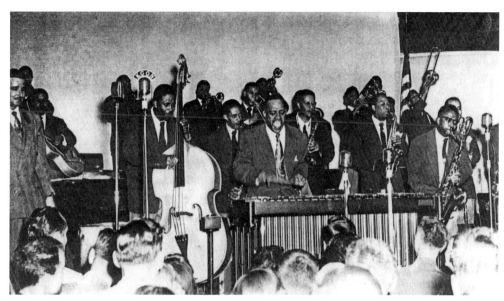

Lionel Hampton and his band live on KGON (courtesy of the author)

Albina Hall and Hibernia Hall. Stanton Duke, Jr. said that he and his dad had no money for advertising, so they made up their own posters and walked all up and down Williams Avenue and then all of the laundry rooms, grocery stores, recreational areas, all over Vanport and Guilds Lake, where many of the Black defense workers were living. "My dad was real close to Lionel Hampton. In fact, Lionel Hampton's my godfather," says Duke, Jr..[10] Stanton Duke met Hampton in the late twenties when he came here with Paul Howard, a territory band out of Los Angeles, with whom Lionel Hampton made some of his first recordings.

Every year for fifteen years, beginning in 1940, Lionel Hampton came to Portland, mostly at McElroy's but also at Jantzen Beach and the Uptown Ballroom. In 1943 he brought in Dinah Washington. In 1946 Hampton whirled into town with two jazz masters of the future, Charles Mingus and Wes Montgomery.

Hampton's opponents accuse him of shameless exhibitionism, of being the ringmaster of a sixteen-man jazz circus. Many forget that some of the most famous jazz musicians passed through the Hampton band and that this man was still playing the vibraphone while he was in his nineties, an instrument that he brought into the realm of jazz in 1930 with a recording by Louis Armstrong. Gunther Schuller, whose observations at times reveal the eyes and ears of a poet, said this: "Hampton's solos tend to be snippets of vibraharp drills or quotes from 'Three Blind Mice'—dopey things— but he plays them with such gusto, such energy, such pyrotechnique, that audiences absolutely go wild."[11]

On July 21, 1949, about two years after Pop McElroy died, Stanton Duke and McElroy's son, Burt, put on the first public interracial dance at the ballroom. Blacks no longer came downtown to dance at McElroy's only on Monday nights. Lionel Hampton and Stanton Duke, in the memory of Pop McElroy, flaunted it in the newspapers and on Sammy Taylor's radio show. At intermission, Hampton's wife, Gladys, took the microphone and announced to the crowd, "It's our big moment when Lionel and I can come to Portland where Lionel first started out with the great Pop McElroy, long before he knew there was a Benny Goodman."[12]

Stanton Duke also did more than his part to advance the cause of women in jazz. He hired a number of female orchestras going back to 1935 with the Harlem Playgirls at the Albina Hall. Later he had the International Sweethearts of Rhythm. Then in 1944 he brought in Eddie Durham's all-girl orchestra.

Duke booked the Floyd Ray territory band with Arnett Cobb and Eddie "Cleanhead" Vinson in 1940. The piano player had been Kenny Bryan, who became a fixture on the Avenue in the mid forties when he and his wife, Marie, were playing with Charlie Merritt. Bryan was a transitional figure, going back and forth between a swing bass in his left hand and the more modern chord forms of Bud Powell.

Trumpeter Erskine Hawkins came to the attention of Portland jazz fans when he played at McElroy's in 1940. Calling himself the twentieth-century Gabriel,[13] Hawkins was a high-note specialist, who apparently liked to punish himself each night by seeing how many high Gs he could hit. His was a band imbued with the blues. It growled and snarled and could sound like Ellington, only dirtier— "the Duke in Dungarees."

Hawkins never had the performers that Duke Ellington had. What he did have was a better dance band. The relaxed beat and big bottom sound of Heywood Henry's baritone saxophone drew thousands of Portlanders to the dance floors of McElroy's and the Uptown Ballroom. Hawkins's recordings sold well in Portland. His "After Hours" was one of the hot selections on the jukebox at Slaughters and one of the reasons Lorraine Walsh Geller wanted to play jazz piano. "Tippin' In" was played almost every night on Bob McAnulty's jazz show for a while and later on became the name of a restaurant.

A little-known jazz secret is that Duke Ellington liked McElroy's so much that he spent two birthdays there, April 29, 1953 and '54. Wally Heider, crack engineer, recorded both events; they are available on a five-volume CD set. When Ellington came through the first time in 1953, a big party for him followed at Bill McClendon's Rhythm Room, where the Duke sat in with a number of local musicians.[14]

Duke Ellington's relationship with Portland goes back to his first appearance at the Heilig Theater in 1933. In May of the next year, *The Oregonian* interviewed Ellington while he was playing at the Mayfair Theater downtown. His fans found out that Ellington didn't like the word jazz. "Negro music is what we are working on," says Ellington, "and you can't play Negro music in a conservatory. This is a music that changes quickly to the extremes of joy and gloom and back again." He was in Portland twice in 1941,

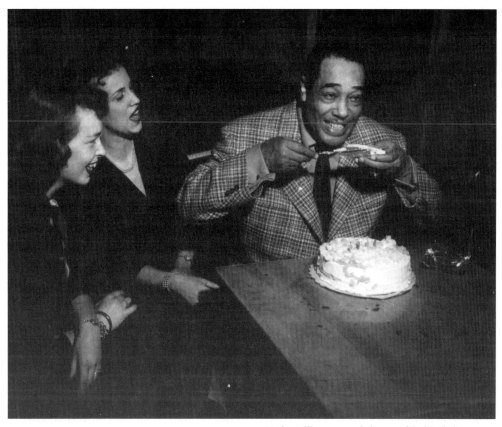

Duke Ellington celebrates his birthday at McElroy's in 1953 (courtesy of McClendon family)

the first time in March and then again in the week following Pearl Harbor in December. He was here again in 1942; he performed and helped sell war bonds at the Victory Center, near where Pioneer Square sits today. Ellington played a concert in August of 1947 at the Civic Auditorium, and Hilmar Grondahl, the high-sounding music critic for *The Oregonian*, wrote this indirect compliment: "Duke Ellington has the potential to make jazz attractive to those who dislike the rum and cola crowd, a crowd who apparently prefer monotonous stomping."[15]

Louis Bellson, Duke Ellington's new percussionist, stunned the crowd at the Civic Auditorium in 1952 with his own composition called "Skin Deep," featuring a five-minute blood-and-thunder drum solo. Everyone in the audience, including the people from RCA Victor, who recorded the band the next night in Seattle, was excited about the way the band was playing. Everyone, that is, except Ted Hallock, who went home and wrote a scathing review that ended up in *Down Beat* under the title "Duke Lays an Egg." Letters in bold defense of Ellington poured in from all over the nation, creating quite a flap for a couple of weeks. Never one for a confrontation, Ellington acted as if it never happened, shrugging it off with something like,

"Well, I guess I'll just have to try a little harder next time when we're in Portland."[16]

In 1970, Ellington and his orchestra paid a visit to Mt. Angel to perform music he had written for Ann Henry, a Portland dancer and choreographer, who was then a resident at Mt. Angel. She had toured with the Ellington Band early in her career. The next year, five hundred well-heeled and dolled-up fans turned out for a dance date at Gracie Hanson's Roaring Twenties in the old Hoyt Hotel, located close to where the Greyhound bus depot is today.[17] In 1973, fronting a band with just a couple of the old names, Duke paid his last visit to Portland, playing to a less than full house at the old Paramount theater, now the Arlene Schnitzer Concert Hall.

One of the biggest surprises at McElroy's in the mid fifties was a group of former Ellington sidemen who had recently left the band and formed a small jazz group under the leadership of Johnny Hodges.[18] The tenor saxophonist was John Coltrane, the man who would become the most influential jazz instrumentalist of the next decade. This was several months before he joined the Miles Davis quintet. In August, just before coming to Portland, the group made a record called "Used To Be Duke," featuring the same personnel that played at McElroy's. Unfortunately there are no solos by John Coltrane.

(All photographs on this page courtesy of Ted Hallock)

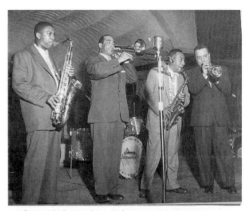

Left to right: John Coltrane, Lawrence Brown, Johnny Hodges, Shorty Baker

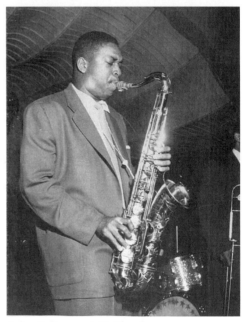

John Coltrane at McElroy's

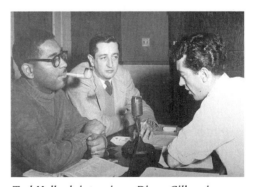

Ted Hallock interviews Dizzy Gillespie while Oregon Journal*'s James Hart looks on*

Benny Carter brought his bus full of boppers in the making to McElroy's on November 15, 1943. Freddy Webster, Curly Russell, and the future poll winner J. J. Johnson were part of the band. Johnson had just recorded his first solo, "Love For Sale," only a few days earlier.[19]

Bop's biggest night at McElroy's happened in February of 1949. Dizzy Gillespie, a goofy-acting, drug-free cofounder of this new music, arrived with his customary goatee, beret, horn-rimmed glasses, and pipe. Many of Portland's leading musicians were there plus most of the members of the Dizzy Gillespie fan club, one of them dressed up to look like Gillespie himself. After all these years the veteran trumpet player Sheldon Brooks still can't believe what he heard that night. "It was the future, right there before us."[20] This was the big band that shook the foundation of Pasadena Center a few months before with their Afro-bop version of "Manteca." This was the band that had recorded Gil Fuller's "Things to Come" a couple of years earlier, a piece so difficult that most bands then and today couldn't cut it. Gillespie and his chief collaborator, Charlie Parker, played Portland in February of 1954 as guest soloists with Stan Kenton. Wally Heider recorded the affair. Part of it appeared on a British LP years ago called *The Definitive Kenton*. It was Parker's last appearance in Portland. Thirteen months later he was dead at thirty-five.

The people's choice at McElroy's Ballroom was Jimmie Lunceford, whose band cut across individual taste like a baby's smile. From 1940 until he died in

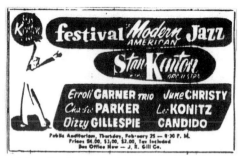

Ad for Charlie Parker's last Portland appearance

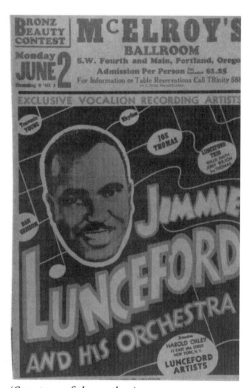

(Courtesy of the author)

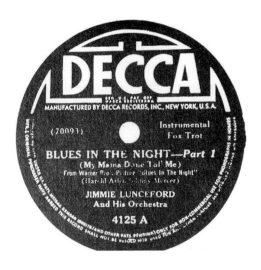

1947, he was in Portland sometimes twice a year, and almost always at McElroy's. Ray Spurgeon recalled how the whole crowd at the ballroom would sigh together when saxophonist Joe Thomas would wind into "Charmaine." Hal Swafford, a very good trombone player in town, who became an even better high school history teacher, was fifteen when he first met Lunceford's trombonist Trummy Young. "I went backstage after hearing them execute some very difficult passage on Lunceford's 'Annie Laurie' and he did it with such nonchalance that I couldn't believe what I heard. When I got backstage, I said, 'How did you do that?' Trummy Young, who was very nice, looked at me and said, 'Page 23 in the Arbans book. You do have the Arban book of trombone exercises, don't you, son?' A quivering 'Yes' came out as I felt the bottom of my jaw hit the ground. See, I thought Black guys just sort of picked it up, and here I am talking to an academic."[21]

Black newspapers in Portland and Seattle played up the fact that Lunceford spoke like a college professor even when he was announcing tunes. They said he had four degrees and that the whole band was composed of college graduates, "forming one of the most intelligent orchestras in pop music," said Seattle's *Northwest Enterprise*.[22] Lunceford softshoed the blues, glossing over the bawdy lyrics, so that even conservative Black people turned out to hear him. (Erskine Hawkins, on the other hand, was out of bounds.) Lunceford's fans loved the cheerful optimism of

songs like "Life is Fine" and "The Best Things in Life are Free." His axiom was "If you've got a style, flaunt it." His greatest arranger, Sy Oliver, took lame songs and made them into catchy hits. It was the way you played it that mattered. No wonder one of the big favorites of the crowds at McElroy's was " 'Tain't What You Do, It's the Way That You Do It." That record and "Blues in the Night," with the great beginning line, "My mama done told me," seemed to be on every hepcat's lips.

The late writer Ralph J. Gleason of the *San Francisco Chronicle* wrote about the effect those Lunceford records had on him in college. "They used to come in on a blue label, thirty-five cents a disc, every couple of weeks at the college bookstore. You had to be on time or the small allotment would be gone and you would have missed the newest Jimmie Lunceford record. If you were lucky enough to get one, you ran back to your room and then you sat back to listen to the sound coming out over your raunchy beatup Magnavox. You savored those records, and since this was long before the economy of abundance and the 78 rpm discs came out one at a time weeks apart, you had time to absorb the records."[23]

Part of the band's appeal was the way they looked: Lunceford in his crisp white suit, waving his baton like a high school drum major, the band in their immaculate bellhop uniforms, the reeds and brass swaying in unison while drummer Jimmy Crawford, sitting in the middle of the battery of shiny hardware, set the dancers in motion. Lunceford died in July 1947, while signing autographs at a record store in Seaside, Oregon, just across the street from the Bungalow, where the band was playing a one-nighter.

Burt McElroy had neither the charisma nor the conviction of his father. Nevertheless he continued to lure in name bands, not just at the ballroom but at the Civic Auditorium. One of his most successful attractions was the Glenn Miller Orchestra under the direction of Tex Beneke. This was a thirty-six-piece unit, equipped with jazz soloists, Jack Sperling and Pete Candoli—one of the great lead trumpet players—Conrad Gozzo, a string section that included Carl Ottobrino from Portland, and five of the best arrangers in the business: Henry Mancini, Bill Finegan, Neal Hefti, Jerry Gray, and a quiet tall former clarinetist and arranger for the Glenn Miller Air Force Band, Norman Leyden. Leyden moved to Portland twenty years later and for thirty-three years has directed the Oregon Pops Concerts, one of the most successful events of the calendar year

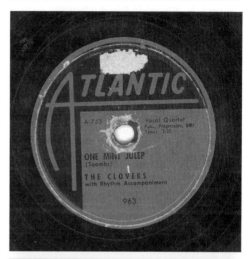

Burton McElroy Presents
Concert
TEX BENEKE
And the 36-Piece
GLENN MILLER
Orchestra
Featuring
Glen Stevens — The Moonlight Serenaders
Jack Sperling — Pete Candoli
Stars of the Chesterfield Supper Club
PUBLIC AUDITORIUM
SUNDAY, FEB. 8 — 8:30 p. m.
Tickets at J. K. Gill Co. — $2.40 - $1.80 - $1.20

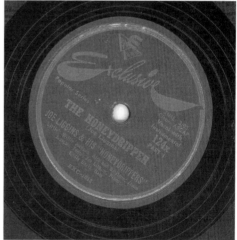

and as close to jazz as many in the audience will ever get.[24]

The truth is that most of the music played at McElroy's and other ballrooms in Portland came from semi-sweet orchestras like the Jerry Van Hoomissen band with little if any jazz arrangements in the book. Pop McElroy's own band, called Cole McElroy's Spanish Ballroom Orchestra, played in the customary dance style of the day, which had nothing to do with jazz.

The breakup of both Black and white big bands gave rise to the popularity of rhythm and blues groups at McElroy's. The favorites were Johnny Moore's Three Blazers, with Oscar Moore on guitar, and the Clovers, a deceptively simple sax and doo-wop sextet that was originally aimed at Black audiences but white middle-class teenagers with money to spend were going batty over "Good Lovin' " and "One Mint Julep."

The incomparable Joe Liggins arrived for a sold-out one-nighter with his Honeydrippers, a name he took from his smash hit.[25] Liggins made a lot of records for the Excelsior label, but nobody remembers anything except for "Honeydripper." It was two sides of a 78 rpm record that could never keep pace with the tremendous demand. Madrona could never keep it in stock, nor could any other record store. Jukebox distributors were going crazy trying to get enough copies, and clubcar porters on the railroad out of L.A. were bootlegging it for ten dollars a copy in Chicago. It's difficult today to understand how a song about a guy with prowess among women could have caused so

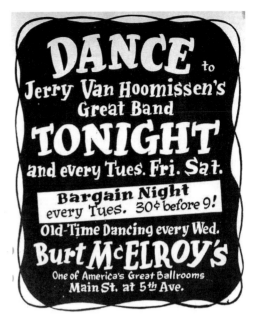

(Courtesy of Margaret Havlicek and Phil Hunt)

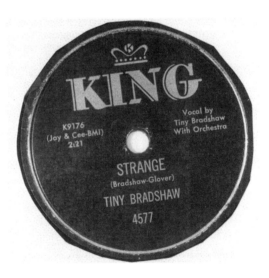

much controversy when it came out in 1945. Some radio stations refused to play it. A restaurant owner asked the distributor to come and take it out of his jukebox because his waitresses were reacting too strongly to the suggestive lyrics. It was interfering with their work.[26]

Of the so-called rhythm and blues groups, Tiny Bradshaw from Youngstown, Ohio, had the most to offer the jazz fans of Portland. Bradshaw was still fronting a jump band stocked with name-brand soloists well into the fifties, long after his contemporaries either had retired or gone completely into rhythm and blues. Bradshaw came to McElroy's many times in the 1940s and '50s, bringing with him some of the stars of the future: Gigi Gryce, Sam Jones, Gil Fuller, Carl Perkins, all of whom praised Bradshaw for the amount of solo time he allowed them.[27]

When the building itself was finally razed in 1980, *The Oregonian* wrote this under the title "McElroy's Last Ball."

The city's favorite annex, 424 SW Main Street, soon to be dust and rubble under the merciless wrecker's ball, will offer a special salute to the wall and floors of yesteryear when the building was once McElroy's Spanish Ballroom. So join us for McElroy's last ball, nostalgia and celebration, with big band music by Bobby Baker's Good Time Band on Sunday, April 20, 1980, 7:00 - 11:00. And in the McElroy's tradition Coca-Cola and Seven-Up will be served. Five dollars a couple. $2.75 singles. Oh, PS: shoulder pads and suspenders welcome.

CHAPTER 14

Uptown Ballroom: "Let Me Off Uptown"

Of the many ballrooms in the Portland area between 1942 and 1957, three stand out for their contribution to the story of jazz—McElroy's, the Golden Canopied Ballroom at Jantzen Beach, and the Uptown Ballroom, formerly known as Dahoney's. The Uptown was a two-story building on the corner of 21st and West Burnside, just down from the Ringside Restaurant. A parking lot and strip mall sit there presently. As at McElroy's, the ballroom was on the second floor, where there was more than a slight echo whenever the trumpet sections blew all out. The best of the big bands came to

the Uptown. One of the earliest was that of Les Hite, who had just taken over from Paul Howard and was featuring a young drummer named Lionel Hampton. Glen Gray and his Casa Loma Orchestra stopped by, playing "No Name Jive" and featuring the astounding clarinet technique of Clarence Hutchinrider.[1]

Prime time at the Uptown was from October 1940 to the middle of '42. The house band was that of Woody Hite, no relation to Les. Woody Hite had to disband in 1942 when most of his sidemen were either being drafted or going to work in the Kaiser shipyards.

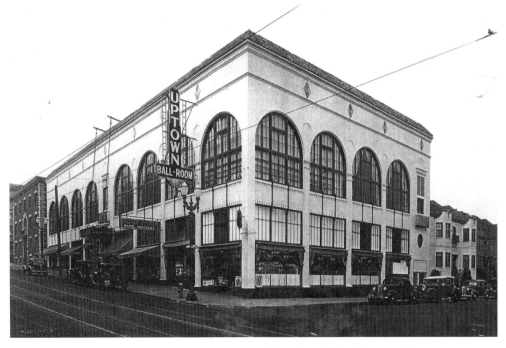

(Courtesy of Ray Spurgeon)

The Woody Hite band resumed thirty years later, thanks to the efforts of Bobby Baker and three of the band's original members—Woody's brother Don, Ray Spurgeon, and Ralph Rosenlund. It's still going in 2005, still serving as a gestation period and springboard for many of Portland's most talented musicians, not to mention a showcase for some of the city's best vocalists, from Jeanne Hackett and Sue Beacock to Shirley Nanette and Rebecca Kilgore. Kilgore, a singer in the school of Doris Day, is the vocalist on the band's only album, *Sentimental Swing*.

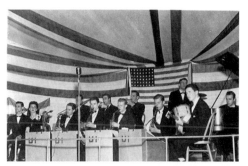

Woody Hite band with Tommy Todd, piano, and Dick Knight, tenor (courtesy of Earl Whitney)

One of the band's high-water marks was the tenor battle that took place New Year's Eve, 1982, at the Marriott Hotel. Sam Schlichting, in a Charlie Ventura state of mind, won a split decision from Tigard's Kenny Hing, on leave from the Count Basie Band. Another memorable night was the benefit for Walter Bridges in 1983. The band roared and stomped as if they had something to prove to the many disc jockeys, broadcasters, and musicians who helped fill the Esquire Club on that November evening. Standouts were Sam Schlichting again, Jeff Uusitalo's bop trombone, and the mighty trumpets of Larry Morrell and Chuck Bradford.[2]

The Hite band wouldn't be alive today without the enthusiasm and dedication of Don Hite, Woody's brother, and the late lead saxophonist, Ray Spurgeon. Spurgeon was only a year out of high school when he joined the Woody Hite band, and has been its de facto chief ever since. Spurgeon was a stockbroker who would rather be playing lead alto in a big band. His job was to blend the

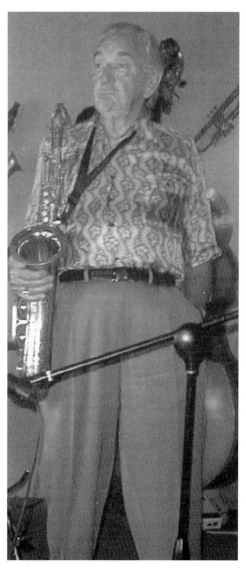

Sam Schlichting, 2005 (courtesy of Ray Spurgeon)

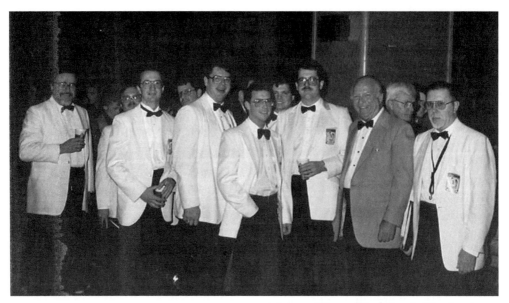

A later edition of the Woody Hite band.
Don Hite is third from the right, tan jacket.
(Courtesy of Hal Swafford)

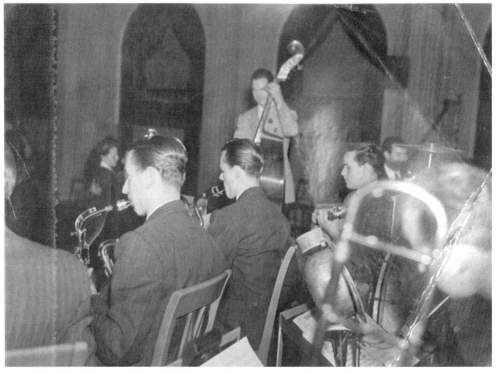

Woody Hite band at the Uptown, 1941
(courtesy of Ray Spurgeon)

saxophones into a cohesive sound, by showing other members how to phrase and articulate according to the arrangement. It's a risky and misunderstood role. That is why there are so many fine soloists on the alto saxophone but few great lead alto players. Ron Hite (no relation), Lee Mack, and of course Ray Spurgeon are the best. Not only must you be aggressive and yet musically sensitive, but you have to have a finely tuned and well-centered tone, one which can pull a saxophone section into harmonic gear.

Ray Spurgeon feels fortunate to have been one of the first of the many "Vancouver Whiz Kids." In an interview some years ago, he talked about his early days at Vancouver High School. "I started as a freshman in 1934, and before that the shop teacher was the band director. And then Chester Duncan came in and he was the one who apparently convinced the board to spend a lot of money on music. People think that Vancouver's reputation for having a great music department started with Wally Hanna. It really started with Chester Duncan, way back when I was a freshman." Spurgeon started on the clarinet under the watchful eye of Eddie Flenner, who was to the future reed students in Portland what Gene Confer was to the prospective piano students. In an interview in a newspaper some years ago, Spurgeon said that he never missed an opportunity to see all the great bands when they came to McElroy's, the Uptown, or Jantzen Beach. One of the personalities who made the biggest impression on him was saxophonist Al Giodello with Paul Whiteman's band, when they came here in 1938. Another memorable experience was at McElroy's in October of 1943 when Benny Carter came through with J. J. Johnson and Freddie Webster. "That five-man saxophone section that Benny had played so beautifully behind his embellishments. They made all the nuances and accents that make standing in front of the bandstand the highlight of the whole evening."

Seeing Duke Ellington at the Uptown in 1941, however, was the most exhilarating experience of Spurgeon's early musical career.

We were the home band at the Uptown at that time so the whole Woody Hite band was there for the Ellington performance. I remember Don Hite went around and got autographs. I think he still has them. Trumpeter Ray Nance had just joined the band and was trying out a new Harmon mute. When he hit the first note on 'Take the A Train,' it popped out and onto the floor and everybody started laughing. At intermission I got to talk to Barney Bigard and that was a lift for me. I remember Jimmy Blanton, the bass player, getting the spotlight, which I'd never seen happen to a bass player before. He was even better in person than on the recordings. Herb Jeffries was doing the singing, wowing the ladies with 'Flamingo.' Ivie Anderson sang her big hit, 'Don't Mean a Thing If It Ain't Got That Swing.' Afterwards, all of us went to the Clover Club downtown, where Blanton and Ben Webster got on the stand and played a duet while the house band, the Russ Graham combo, looked on in bewilderment. No one had ever imagined a bass violin could be played as if it were a wind instrument.

Of the many versions of the Woody Hite band, Ray Spurgeon still favors the original 1941 group, despite the fact that the war had taken many of the best sidemen. The brains behind the band at the time belonged to arranger and composer Milt Kleeb. "He had a real knack for voice leading," says Spurgeon. "The way he could blend the saxes and the trumpets into a single line was truly amazing." Sixty years later some of those

arrangements are still in the Hite book. Kleeb was so far ahead of his time that he became one of the arrangers of the most farsighted orchestra of that time, Boyd Raeburn's. Kleeb's composition "Boyd's Nest," based on Charlie Parker's "Bird's Nest," was a favorite with members of the Raeburn band, which at various times included Dizzy Gillespie and Lucky Thompson. But even the best arranger in the Northwest wouldn't have been able to swing the Woody Hite band if it didn't have the talent. The 1941-'42 Uptown group had a huge amount. The quality of the personnel outweighed the constant turnover, especially after Pearl Harbor. Tommy Todd was doing some of

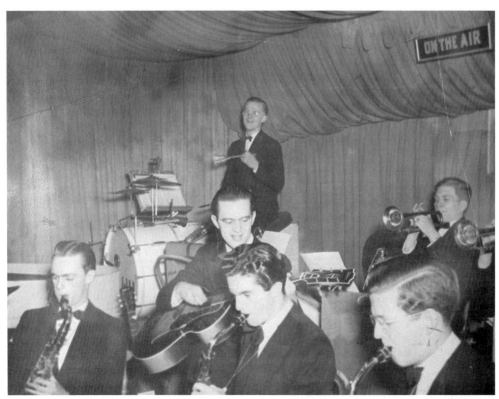

Warren Black on guitar; in front, on his left, saxophonist Milt Kleeb; next to Kleeb is saxophonist Ray Spurgeon (courtesy of Virginia Black)

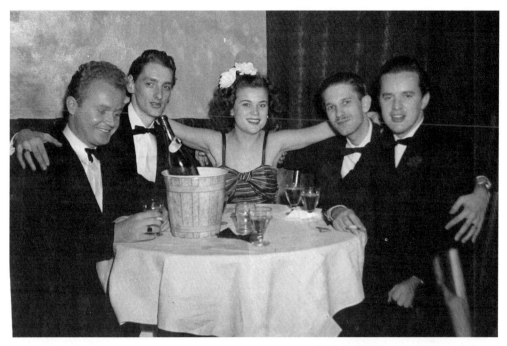

Warren Black cocktail table. Left to right: Al Carter, Russ Hackett, Jeannie Hackett, unknown, Warren Black (courtesy of Virginia Black)

the writing and playing piano; Don Norlander, a skinny kid with a tremendous range, who could nail high G's with the utmost ease, was on trumpet. Also on trumpet was Francis Shirley, one of the magnificent Shirley sisters, who went on to play with Charlie Barnet. Jay Dreyer was playing trumpet with his amazing technique. The Harry James of the Woody Hite band was Bob Sigafoos, and the beat was maintained by the energetic Al Carter on drums and Woody Hite, the leader of the band, on bass.[3]

One unique member of the Woody Hite original band was Warren Black, the fun-loving father of electric guitar in Portland. Black was the first Portlander to bring jazz guitar to the foreground. He was the first to give it a place and a voice

equal to the trumpet or the saxophone, and the first in town with the latest chords: the augmented and diminished chords that his mentor, Charlie Christian, was using with Benny Goodman when they played at Jantzen Beach in 1939. Warren Black was the first to put out a book of the basic chord changes to most of the frequently requested pop songs, a book that is still being used in Portland and has been sighted as far away as Tokyo. In short, Black is the beginning of a line of guitar players that extends from Ernie Hood to Buddy Fite to Michael Denny, all the way to the contemporary designs of Ralph Towner and Dan Balmer. Warren Black's solo on "I Can't Give You Anything But Love," from a broadcast by the Woody Hite band in 1941, shows how far ahead he was.

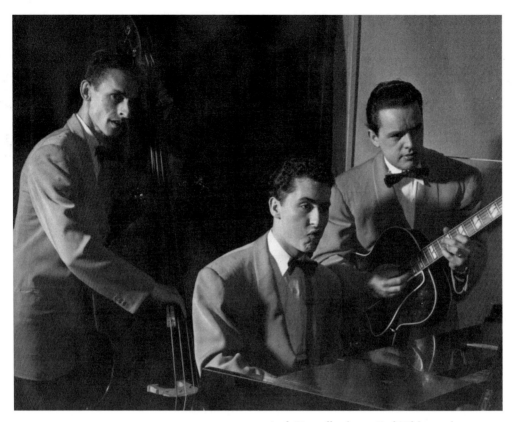

Jack Howell, piano; Earl Whitney, bass; Warren Black, guitar (courtesy of Virginia Black)

Black's favorite playing partner at the Uptown and elsewhere was Jack Howell, a thirty-year veteran of Portland nightclubs, twenty of those years behind the piano at the London Grill in the Benson Hotel. Their repertoire was infinite. Hardly a published tune existed to which they didn't know the words and chords. "He had a personality that could make a musical hack feel like an innovative genius," commented one of Howell's friends. Howell was fifty-one when he died in 1976. His name still comes up, though, whenever the conversation turns to the premier pianists of Portland.

Another student in the Charlie Christian school of guitar was Glen Parker, a bespeckled, mustachioed man from White Salmon, Washington. Parker couldn't read music, probably never made a commercial record, and it's doubtful that five people would even remember when he used to sit in with Herbie Hall at Bill's Gold Coin just across the street from the Uptown Ballroom. Hall's piano brought out the best in Parker, and with Bob Douglass and Dick Hall on bass and drums, this was one of the better quartets of the time.[4]

The Uptown Ballroom became the Palais Royale in the late forties and

straight bands became the policy. One of
the exceptions was Vido Musso, Stan
Kenton's he-man tenor saxophonist on
"Come Back to Sorrento" and "Artistry
Jumps," two reasons why Kenton was
topping the jazz polls in the 1940s. A
built-in audience of mostly Kenton
crazies was waiting for Musso when he
arrived for a two-night stand. Imagine
the look on their faces when they learned
that Musso's new band was trying to
copy Benny Goodman, the King of Swing.
Not Benny Goodman, 1951, but Benny
Goodman, 1936, when most of the
people in the audience that night had
been in grade school. Everywhere that
Musso went, the ghost of Kenton
followed. So after diminishing
attendance and luke-warm reviews,
Musso gave it up. His loyal fans would
have to wait five years for a reunion of
Stan Kenton and Vido Musso.[5]

CHAPTER 15

Jantzen Beach: "Dancin' at Jantzen"

Interstate I-5 takes you within a couple of hundred yards of where the Golden Canopied Ballroom at Jantzen Beach used to be. It was part of a huge amusement complex that could boast of a historic merry-go-round, a heart-stopping roller-coaster, and the West Coast's second-largest swimming pool, built to sell Jantzen swimwear. You take that exit now, the one just before you cross the Interstate Bridge, and all you will find is a shopping mall. The only reminder of yesteryear is the clock on top of Waddles Restaurant.

When Sam Donahue finished playing "Goodnight Ladies" on September 13, 1957, the music stopped, ending thirty years and more than a thousand nights of "dancin' at Jantzen." No one was more dejected than the ballroom's manager, Sam Amato. The big bands had stopped coming to the point that, to make ends meet, Amato had had to hire rockabilly stars like Gene Vincent and his Blue Caps. And so the canopied ballroom, like so many other ballrooms that were an integral part of amusement parks, became a bowling alley. The demise of big bands can be traced all the way back to the shortages of World War II and by the late fifties only a few were still touring. Amato, in an interview in 1982, said, "People keep asking me when the bands are coming back. But what are they coming back to? Television and Elvis Presley ruined it in the 1950s."[1]

The short, stocky, Amato is highly talkative, and is Portland's star witness to the swing era. He opened the Jantzen Beach Ballroom in the late twenties playing drums with Don DeForest. Hank Wales was on bass. In 1934 Amato backed the future pinup queen, Betty Grable, at the old Orpheum Theater downtown. When he was with Archie Loveland in 1939, Judy Garland was the singer. He's traded drum choruses with Gene Krupa in New York. His proudest moment was the night when the great drummer Sid Catlett asked (maybe in jest) if Amato would give him a few lessons. "Geez," says Amato, "I told him I should be taking from you. Oh, I don't know, maybe he liked my tom-tom work on Sherwood's 'Elk's Parade.' You know, I had Bobby Sherwood's big band in when I ran Jantzen Beach. I had good technique. My cousin Joe Amato was a national rudiment drum champion and went on to play with the Portland Symphony. The guy I tried to copy was George Marsh, with Paul Whiteman. Geez, Whiteman had a band. Of course, he could afford to pay the highest wages. I stood right in front of him. It was at McElroy's and I watched Marsh, and Bing

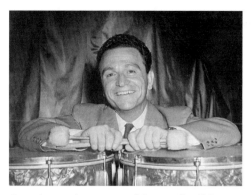

Sam Amato (courtesy of Amato family)

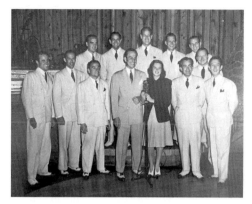

Judy Garland with Archie Loveland
(courtesy of Amato family)

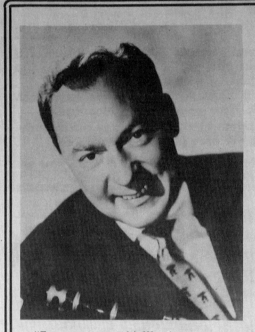

SAMMY AMATO
presents

WOODY HERMAN

and his new

Third Herd

featuring

DOLLY HOUSTON

and fourteen
Top Instrumentalists

— 5 NIGHTS —
AUGUST 3-4-5-6-7

dancing from 9 p. m. to 1 a. m.
in the
golden canopied ballroom

JANTZEN BEACH
TW 5555

"Forty-one-year-old Woodrow Wilson (Woody) Herman was back in town—and back on top of the musical heap—with his Third Herd, the most versatile band he has ever lead."
(from Time magazine)

Vancouver Bus . . . Hiway 99 near Interstate Bridge

(Courtesy of Margaret Havlicek and Phil Hunt)

Crosby, who had just joined him and had a big bandage across his head. I forget where they were staying now. Crosby had just been in an accident with two other singers that were part of that famous trio."[2]

Amato was also in the front row at McElroy's when the jazz giant Fats Waller and his sextet played there in July of 1941. "Oh it was hot. Geez, only about one hundred people showed up 'cause it was 104 degrees and no air conditioning, all those hot sweaty people. Many went out to the parking lot and listened to the music coming through the window. I was there with the band leader Jerry Van Hoomissen whom I was playing with at the time. Margaret Carrol was singing, as I remember. It was a very good dance band, no jazz, but very good dance band. Jerry and I went out to the parking lot with the rest of them and listened to the whole thing while people around us were dancing."[3]

Jantzen Beach Ballroom in its time hosted hundreds of big bands and most of them played little if any Jazz. Yet when the dance date was over, there always seemed to be one or two sidemen looking to sit in someplace like Paul's Paradise or the Chicken Coop. "We were always learning from those cats coming through town," trumpeter Bobby Bradford once said. Many were coming from the ballrooms like the Uptown, McElroy's, and Jantzen Beach. Not that there weren't plenty of big bands that would be classified as jazz. Woody Herman brought in his Second Herd in 1949, the one with Stan Getz. In August of '54 his Third Herd arrived, with those wrought-iron bandstands, the great arrangements of Ralph Burns, and a surefire drummer named Chuck Flores. Thanks again to Wally Heider, a CD is available of that balmy night fifty years ago.

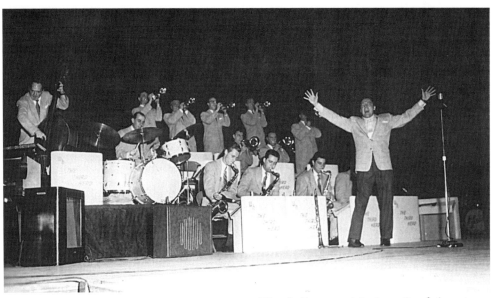

Woody Herman at Jantzen Beach (courtesy of Ted Hallock)

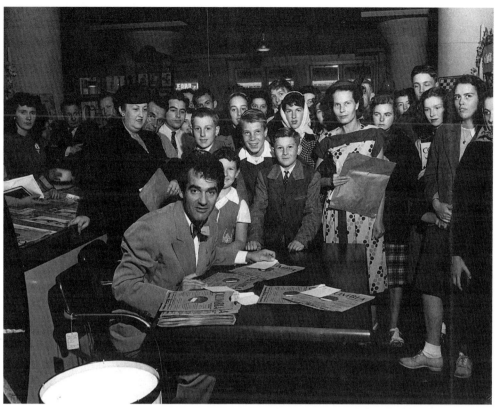

Gene Krupa and fans (courtesy of Ted Hallock)

America's number-one drummer played a three-day engagement at Jantzen Beach Ballroom in March of 1946, introducing the arranging talents and baritone saxophone of Gerry Mulligan. It was Gene Krupa who brought the drums to center stage with his famous solo on "Sing, Sing, Sing" at Benny Goodman's Carnegie Hall concert in 1938. Krupa's appeal was more than his technique or his ability to swing when top-notch white drummers were scarce. He was fascinating to watch, every move a picture. Krupa was Slingerland Drum Company's poster boy, a gyrating, gum-chewing, tousle-haired forerunner to Elvis Presley. He had legions of fans of both sexes, many of whom showed up at Jantzen Beach and/or at J. K. Gill's on Saturday waiting in line to get his autograph or better yet a pair of his drum sticks. Portland authority on Gene Krupa, Steve Brockway, talked about his meeting as if he were encountering the Dalai Lama. "I wanted a pair of sticks so badly that when my turn came in line, I couldn't stop myself from asking him for his sticks, and can you believe that he reached down in his bag and gave them to me? That was over fifty years ago. They are still hanging in a velvet case in my closet."[4]

Fresh out of Balboa Beach, California, and anxious to test his popularity, Stan Kenton played his first job on the road at Jantzen Beach. He got stranded in

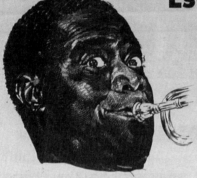

SAMMY AMATO presents . . .

LOUIS ARMSTRONG

and the

Esquire All-Stars

featuring

☆ Velma Middleton ☆

☆ Trummy Young ☆

☆ Barney Bigard ☆

☆ Arvell Shaw ☆

☆ Billy Kyle ☆

LOUIS 'SATCHMO' ARMSTRONG

- An inspired singer
- The world's greatest trumpet player
- Born in New Orleans 54 years ago, he has set the pattern for the development of American jazz.

—— One Night Only ——

SAT., OCT. 23

dancing in the
Golden Canopied Ballroom
9 P.M. to 1 A.M.

JANTZEN BEACH

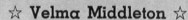

(Courtesy of Margaret Havlicek and Phil Hunt)

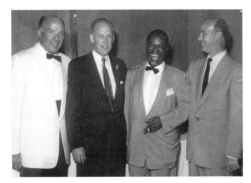

Louis Armstrong with Portland mayor Terry Schrunk, flanked by the Amato brothers (courtesy of Amato family)

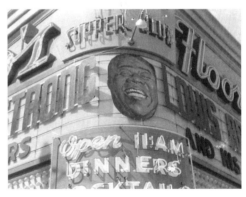

(Courtesy of Amato family)

Portland for two weeks, and stayed at the Joyce Hotel, which still stands at SW 11th and Stark, just above the Fish Grotto restaurant.[5]

Louis Armstrong was very popular with the dancers at the Golden Canopied Ballroom. In 1943 he was here as part of a World War II Victory Drive to sell bonds. In 1944 he had a birthday in Portland. For the next eight years he played at Amato's, McElroy's, and the Auditorium, but mostly at Jantzen Beach, a fact that did not sit well with certain civil rights advocates, who objected to the segregated policy there.[6]

Some say Louis Armstrong played Portland so often because he was crazy about the food at Myrtle Barno's gumbo restaurant on NE Broadway, or maybe it was the scrumptious sweet potatoes and barbecue at Nance's.[7] Sometimes Armstrong would stay with his close friend Monte Ballou of the Castle Jazz Band, whose attic at one time was filled with rare Armstrong memorabilia. It was Monte Ballou who discovered two of Armstrong's recordings thought to be lost, "Lulu's Ball" and "Workingman's Stomp," records he found in the bottom of a barrel in a junk shop.

Armstrong came to town in 1949 with Jack Teagarden.[8] Teagarden was Louis Armstrong's counterpart on trombone. Teagarden, Miff Mole, and Jimmy Harrison were the pioneers of swing trombone in the 1920s. Teagarden played the canopied ballroom for six straight years and was well known for picking up Portland musicians and taking them on the road. Lee Rockey, George Bruns, and Francis Shirley's sister Mildred were all in the band for a short period.

The best-known Portlander to play with Teagarden was the popular Freddie Keller, a trombone player himself and an important member of the Teagarden band. Armed with a book of Milt Kleeb arrangements inherited from the defunct Hite band of 1942, Keller became the crowd favorite at Jantzen Beach. He never sounded better than he did a couple of days before Christmas in 1960 at Meier and Frank's in Salem.[9] Behind the bold and insistent drumming of Dave Longtin Jr., Keller turned a dance date into a jazz recital. Standout soloists were Jim Smith on trumpet, Quen Anderson, and tenor saxophonist Gene Zarones, whose distilled tone and fluid drive caught the ear of name-band leader Les Elgart, who hired Zarones for a coast-to-coast tour.

"Zarones had the soul of a Robin Williams," says fellow bandmate Dan Mason, "and Freddie Keller loved insanity, so even if he had a full sax section he would hire Zarones on piano just to watch him cut up—maybe playing a solo while sitting on top of the piano or stuffing a banana down the throat of Keller's trombone. He might throw a towel over his arm and play the role of a waiter going table to table taking orders. One time at the Way Out, he put on a chef hat, went out to the kitchen, and made sandwiches out of dollar bills."[10]

In high school, Gene Zarones was a sixty-minute football player in the days before face guards, when a stiff arm to the mouth was not uncommon and could

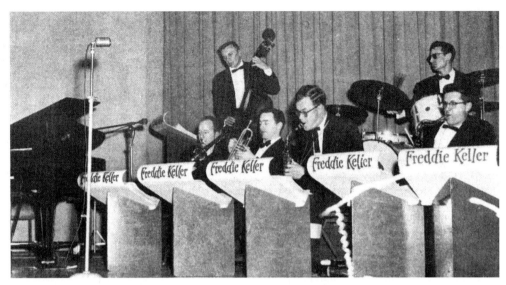

*Freddie Keller and his group, 1959
(courtesy of the author)*

have cost him his career. He survived that to become, at least for a while, the toast of Portland's big-band tenors. Unfortunately he did not survive a crash in the late sixties while flying his own airplane over the Tillamook Forest just weeks after receiving his pilot's license.

Freddie Keller always seemed to have the best trombone section in town. Maybe it's because he played the instrument himself. Not just the stand-out soloists but solid ensemble players such as John Trudeau, Gary Nelson, and future band leader George Reinmiller, a former Portland Symphony member, whose bands were very much in the Woody Hite tradition, sometimes using many of the same personnel.

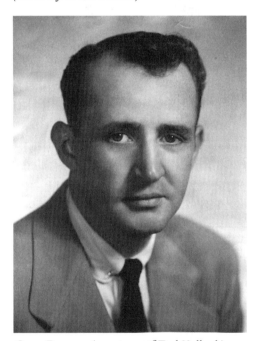

Gene Zarones (courtesy of Ted Hallock)

Keller's most famous trombone player was Rod Levitt, the triple threat from Grant High School. Levitt hasn't played jazz for a living since 1966, after he had made the last of four octet records in New York, three of them for RCA Victor. The *New York Times* and *Down Beat* had

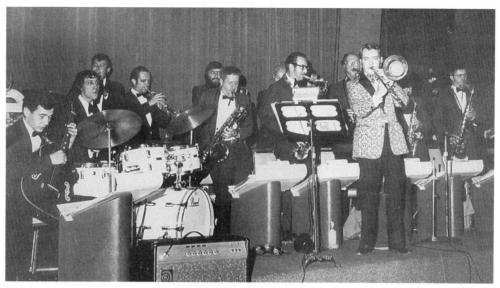

George Reinmiller band (courtesy of Hal Swafford)

some flattering things to say about this rollicking group of nobodies.[11] John S. Wilson, the Pauline Kael of jazz, was one of the toughest critics in the early sixties. Only a handful of records received his highest rating. Two of them were by Levitt's octet: *Dynamic Sound Patterns* on Riverside and *Insight* on RCA Victor. Listen to what Wilson had to say about Levitt's *Insight* album from 1965. "Things happen, all kinds of things, in solos, in ensembles, and this band rides hard and generates a kind of excitement and sense of originality dressed in full professionalism that is scarcely ever expected in jazz anymore."[12] More than that, Albert McCarthy and a number of British jazz authorities believe that these octet recordings rank with the very best of their kind.

The title *Insight* was named after a special events program on KATU-TV. It was hosted by Doug Ramsey, now a well-known jazz writer and personal friend of Rod Levitt. Levitt's favorite on that album is "The Mayor of Vermont Village." "I wrote that for my Dad," says Levitt. "Vermont Village is a community in southwest Portland and my folks were the first residents. So I used to call him the Mayor of Vermont Village."[13]

Levitt is about six foot tall and looks like he may have wrestled or played a little football. And what his pals saw at Grant High School in 1948 is about what you see today. Still the same wide-eyed enthusiasm over the simple things in life, like homemade pie and ice cream. " One of the best things about living," Levitt says.

My brother got me into jazz. He was taking piano from Gene Confer and got me excited. The first trombone player I heard was Lawrence Brown, with Duke Ellington, and then later I heard Bill Harris play "I Surrender, Dear" on the radio, with Woody Herman. At Grant

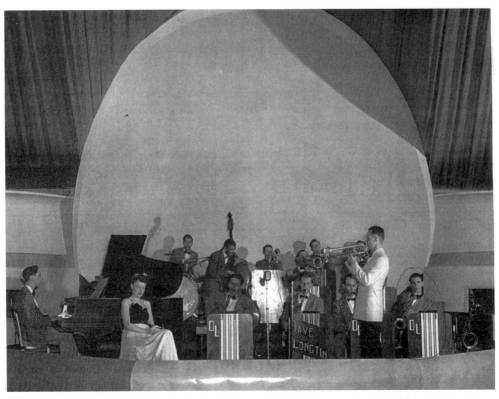

Dave Longtin, Sr., with Rod Levitt (courtesy of Hal Swafford)

High School we founded a group with Ron Hite on sax and Jerry Magill on bass. We called ourselves the Mad Lepers. We had sweatshirts and Dizzy Gillespie berets. We were quite taken with Charlie Parker and Dizzy Gillespie. I still have some acetate tapes of those days. Also I was playing with Dave Longtin, Sr., and his orchestra gave me a lot of experience. I was with Freddie Keller at Jantzen Beach. That was a very good band with Sam Schlichting on tenor, and then I was jamming at the Coop a lot, whenever I could, learning from people like Sid Porter, Eddie Wied, and a guy with very good ideas that I'd totally forgotten about, Hal Koster. I remember the night Lorraine Walsh came into the club and just tore the place up.[14]

In Portland, Rod Levitt was a sideman with Monte Ballou and the Castle Jazz Band. It was one of his most valuable experiences. He learned the techniques and tricks that would later come in handy with his own octet. In the Castle Jazz Band, solos were just bridges between the ensembles. The sound of the whole group was more important than any one virtuoso. "I fell into their sound right away. I still love that kind of music although they didn't want me at first. I was taking George Bruns' place when he went to California, and everybody in the band felt I was too modern. What they played was really authentic stuff and they were really good players who could play with a lot of fire. There was Freddy Crew and Bob Short and I will tell you, those tunes aren't easy, like 'Ory's Creole Trombone.' People who don't play that kind of music don't understand."[15]

After a short time at Reed College, Levitt left for the University of Washington, where he met the famous Quincy Jones, a contact that would later get him an invitation to Dizzy Gillespie's big band in 1956. The Gillespie band went on a goodwill tour that year. Levitt didn't get many solos with that band because everywhere he looked there was some future Hall of Famer: Lee Morgan, Wynton Kelly, Benny Golson, Phil Woods, to name a few. He did get to the Middle East, courtesy of the State Department, where he and the rest of the Gillespie band played jazz to millions of people who had never heard it before. Three albums came out of this tour, *Dizzy in Greece, Dizzy World Statesman,* and *Birk's Works.*

In 1958, Levitt appeared on a Gil Evans record called *Great Jazz Standards* and not long after that he was playing with the Gerry Mulligan big band. This was before he landed his most lucrative job, in the trombone section of the Radio Music Hall Orchestra. And that is where the idea of the octet came to him. Levitt says,

The idea of the octet was to find eight very good musicians from the Music Hall or elsewhere who were as bored with studio work as I was and who would be willing to rehearse some very challenging material on their own time. We rehearsed all of the tunes on Dynamic Sound Patterns *for two years before we felt ready to make a record. While the*

critics loved us when we played at the Newport Jazz Festival, I never made a dime with that group. The records never sold. Nobody wanted to hire us. What was I going to do with an eight-piece band that doesn't play the standards? So, I gave it up. Do I wish I could have written for those guys forever? Sure, but I had a family. I am now in the business of making commercials and jingles. I still play once in a while. There have been some reunions of the octet. But I am not a jazz musician any more. Not the way I was when I was playing with Freddie Keller at Jantzen Beach and jamming afterwards at the Coop with Dick Knight. Those days are long gone.[16]

But not forgotten. Thirty-five years ago a book came out called *Jazz on Record,* a guide to the recordings that best illustrate the development of jazz from 1917 to 1967. Rod Levitt's *Dynamic Sound Patterns* was one of the albums mentioned.[17]

One of Levitt's biggest fans is Portland composer/pianist, Dave Frishberg.

Recently I listened to the Rod Levitt RCA and Riverside recordings that I first heard forty years ago. Today it seems to me that Levitt, besides being a master orchestrator, was the most melodic, the most audacious, the most colorful, the wittiest, and the most engaging jazz composer of the time. Like Ellington, he writes with the listener in mind, and like Ellington, he leads the listener around by the ear. Levitt's way with jazz is thoughtful without being subtle. It's very Ellingtonian at times. But Levitt's personal humor and intelligence are what

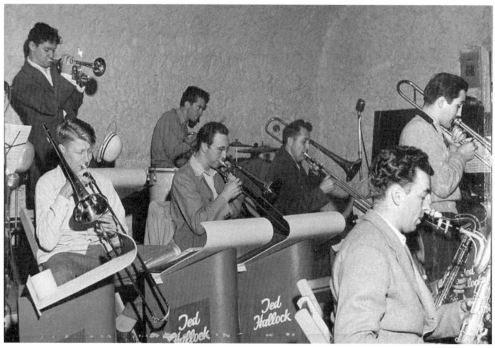

Ted Hallock orchestra, Wally Heider on baritone saxophone in the foreground (courtesy of Ted Hallock)

chime through everything. And what a band he put together for these recordings. These forty-year-old recordings still sound fresh today, and I think it is because Levitt produced meticulously detailed music of the highest order and sophistication and entrusted it to these carefully selected players who responded heroically. I think Levitt's name belongs on a list that includes Ellington, Strayhorn, Ralph Burns, Bill Holman, and a handful of other elitely accomplished and profound composers who happen to be jazz players.[18]

Keller's competition at Jantzen Beach in the early forties was the totally forgotten Kenny Baker band. It was an all-white West Coast territory band stationed out of California. They played in the manner of Benny Goodman. Baker traveled up and down the West Coast before settling in Portland in about 1939. His sidemen included Tommy Todd, the Hood brothers, Bob Steiner, Bill DeSousa from Salem, and Milt Kleeb, when Baker was able to lure him away from Woody Hite. Altoist Marty Wright, who was in the band for a while, says that tenor Zoot Sims joined the band when they were in California, and that's where he got his nickname, when someone arbitrarily put "Zoot" on the front of his music stand. The name stayed with him for the rest of his life.[19]

Ted Hallock also had a loyal following at Jantzen Beach. He returned from World War II, enrolled at the University of Oregon in 1946, and put together a band that played all over the state, especially at Jantzen Beach. Gene Zarones was the outstanding soloist and future recording engineer Wally Heider was on baritone. Hallock was the drummer. "We chartered a Greyhound bus like the big shots," Hallock says. "Only problem was it gave my sidemen a sort of traveling club house to drink in." Hallock left the band in November 1947, and moved to Chicago to become assistant editor for *Down Beat.* He offered his players the band's book, stands, uniforms, etc., free, to carry on the orchestra. "They didn't have the spirit or the guts to accept," Hallock muses.[20]

Sammy Amato has his own favorites: Harry James, all of the Glenn Miller-styled orchestras that included Jerry Gray, Ralph Flanagan, Tex Beneke. Says Amato,

'Course I'd have to say, if we are talking about money, Guy Lombardo outdrew everyone. There must have been 4300 in the ballroom and Jantzen Beach Ballroom was the biggest ballroom in town. The biggest egg laid out there was the Sauter and Finegan Concert Orchestra. Now I am not saying it wasn't great music, but the dancers just stood around like it was a circus act or something.

I had Les Brown in the mid fifties. Geez, they could do everything, novelty stuff, ballads, jazz. I booked them in as a dance band and a lot of people came expecting that it was going to be that. Instead they were standing thirty feet deep listening to a jazz concert. Geez, the drummer he had. Les had his own sound.[21]

Forty years later in an interview just hours before his last performance in Portland, at the Hilton Hotel, Les Brown referred to it as the "Sound of Renown." "It is very difficult to get an original sound, and I wanted something that would immediately identify our band, so I went to Frank Comstock, our main arranger, and with a little help from me, he basically came up with the idea of Harmon mutes, a trombone choir, and the guitar on top. You can hear it on our ballads."[22]

Portlanders heard more of Les Brown than any other big band in the last part of the twentieth century. Starting in 1946 he was in Portland almost every year after that. For the first ten years or so, mostly at Jantzen Beach. After that it was the Hoyt Hotel, Civic Auditorium, the Paramount, and Hilton Hotel for eight straight years until 1994. Les Brown is in Ripley's *Believe it or Not* for having the longest-lasting musical organization of the twentieth century. This was made possible in large part because his band was Bob Hope's back-up band for decades. Each summer they toured to San Francisco, Portland, Seattle, and the Midwest. The purpose was to promote their recordings. One recording in particular caught the fancy of disc jockeys Sammy Taylor and Bob McAnulty, and in turn many jazz fans in Portland. It's called *Concert at the Palladium*, a two-record set done around Labor Day in 1953. They were on fire that night, and on the strength of those recordings and the reputation of many of Les Brown's sidemen, *Metronome* voted them Band of the Year in 1955 over the bands led by

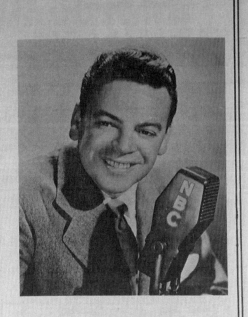

SAMMY AMATO
presents

LES BROWN

and his
BAND OF RENOWN

featuring

JO ANN GREER
BUTCH STONE
STUMPY BROWN
RAY SIMS
DAVE PELL

—— One Night Only ——
FRI., MARCH 25
dancing in the
Golden Canopied Ballroom
9 P. M. to 1 A. M.

JANTZEN BEACH

The Maestro

- Winner of Downbeat's 1954 poll for No. 1 Band of the Year
- Featured on Bob Hope's radio and television shows
- Coral recording artist

(Courtesy of Margaret Havlicek and Phil Hunt)

Stan Kenton, Count Basie, and Duke Ellington. When they came to Portland in March of 1955, Portland fans were waiting for them and Wally Heider, one of Les Brown's most enthusiastic supporters, was there to record them.

Les Brown reluctantly admitted that his '54-'55 editions were his best. Reluctantly because Brown had a reputation as a disciplinarian in the manner of Glenn Miller and Tommy Dorsey. But this was one organization he couldn't control. Some writers were calling it a jazz band masquerading as a dance band. Gunther Schuller in his book *The Swing Era* says that what happened to the Brown band between 1937 and 1955 was one of the biggest transformations in the history of popular or jazz music. "An ugly cocoon to quite a beautiful butterfly." Kenny Hing came away admiring the all-out swing and precision of the band. Ray Spurgeon stood in front of the band for hours listening to every nuance from the pure-toned lead alto saxophone of Ronny

Lang. "We had a chemistry," admits Brown, "and it can't be duplicated. We brought out a Comstock arrangement not too long ago and it sounded terrible. You're never going to get that chemistry again. There have been many big bands when everybody was an all-star and poll winner, but we had the right chemistry between ensemble players and soloists and their two different styles. Where am I going to get another Dave Pell, Tony Rizzi, or a trumpeter like Don Fagerquist, who used to start on a run that would seem to go on forever so that in the middle of the solo I used to yell out, 'Breathe, Don, breathe' or Ray Sims, our trombone player? He played with such heart that even today, forty years later, when I listen to his records, I still get goose bumps."[23]

Another frequent visitor at the Golden Canopied Ballroom was Charlie Barnet. Like Teagarden, he used a number of Portlanders in his band: Fran Shirley, Ernie Hood, Ralph Rosenlund. Ron Hite joined for a while. Barnet's biggest catch from the banks of the Columbia was a boy named Carl or Little Doc in deference to his father, a dentist who had an office in Portland. Barnet hired Carl Severinsen right off the stage at Jantzen Beach. Charlie Barnet tells it this way. "Our first job after the Argent Ballroom was Jantzen Beach in Portland, Oregon. A good friend of mine in the city was Sam Amato. As soon as we arrived he started to pound my ear about a young player he wanted me to hear. Now I'm usually reluctant to have musicians sit in with the band on the job because nine times out of ten it's an absolute disaster. But

Sam kept pushing me until I said OK. I'll let the kid play the last set. The rest is musical history because the trumpet player was Doc Severinsen. I told him to go home, get his clothes, because he was joining the band. He says, 'Well, I don't want to take anybody's job,' and I says, 'You're not. I just added a trumpet player.' "[24]

Seattle has at least two jazz titans: Quincy Jones and Ray Charles. Doc Severinsen is the closest thing Portland has to a big name, and he's from Arlington, Oregon, in cattle ranch and wheat farming country, a hundred and twenty-five miles down the Columbia Gorge. Except for a short stint with Sam Donahue in 1948 and Tommy Dorsey a little later, Doc Severinsen was with Barnet for about three years. Barnet's bop band of 1949 was the most exciting. They came to Jantzen not as a dance band but as one of the best jazz bands, featuring the great drummer/composer Tiny Kahn, and a busload of former Kenton sidemen in the trumpet section. Harry James called them the best trumpet section he ever heard: Maynard Ferguson, Sweden's Rolf Ericson, Ray Wetzel, the husband of Bonnie Wetzel of Vancouver, and Doc Severinsen, who was given solos on "Cuba" and Pete Rugolo's "Overtime."

In a few polls, Doc Severinsen was voted the nation's number-one trumpet player, more for his virtuosity than for his improvisations. Nonetheless, Leonard Feather asked him to represent the United States in an International Bop Sextet recorded on Metro Records. The sextet was made up of some of the finest

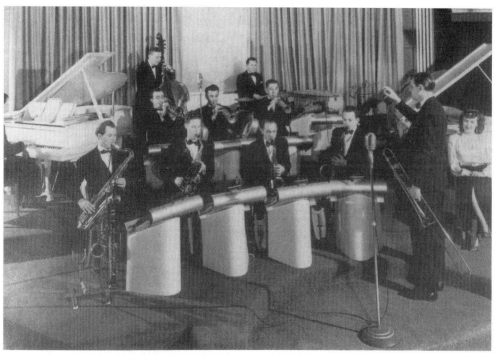

*Doc Severinsen with George Bruns band
(courtesy of Don Proctor)*

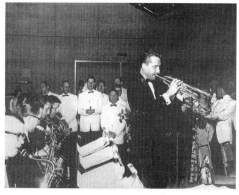

*Doc Severinsen in Portland (courtesy of Hal
Swafford)*

jazz musicians from all over the world.
Japan's Toshiko Akiyoshi was the leader.
Severinsen gives a good account of
himself on "Swingin' till the Girls Come
Home."

On top of all the clinics and recording
that Doc Severinsen did in the 1950s and
'60s, he still managed to get in four
hours of practice a day. In high school he
had won state and national titles on
trumpet. His three models, all of whom
came to Jantzen Beach, were Sonny
Dunham, Harry James, and Dick Mains,
the trumpet player with Teddy Powell.
Not long after Severinsen graduated from
high school, he joined Ted Fiorito. The
drummer in that band was KBOO jazz
broadcaster, Don Manning. Manning
remembers,

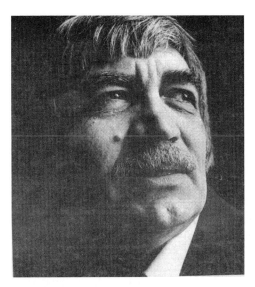

Don Manning (courtesy of Tim Jewett)

I joined Fiorito in Seattle, where I was living at the time. The next day we went to Portland and the trumpet player we had in the band quit. Now in those days, which was near the end of World War II, we were still fighting hard. It was about 1944, and the only guys that were available were the ones who were 4-F, or children or women. Well, the next day they bring in this child prodigy, this little kid with a cornet. We're all looking over our music. I'm looking over the drum music and over there in a corner by himself, just blasting away on his warm-ups, is Doc Severinsen. And even then you could tell this kid means business. He was about sixteen, I guess, and already he wants to play lead trumpet.

Naturally some of the guys in the band don't like it. They're sayin' things like 'Oh God, robbing the cradle!' and 'What's next?' but then Ted Fiorito is very cool and a pretty good piano player, who at that time was converting his hotel band to a swing band. He gets up in front of us

and says, 'Hey, let's give the kid a shot, OK?' and everybody in the band starts to grumble. So then Severinsen starts in on 'Melancholy Baby,' which later became his feature number. Well, he had so much power and he played it up, down, and backwards, and you couldn't help but be impressed. Well, Fiorito just flipped out, ecstatic, he couldn't go to sleep from thinking about how this kid was going to be a big star and a big drawing card for the band. Well, some of the guys liked him but some of the older guys were saying that he wasn't even playing jazz, as great as it sounded. They said he was just doing exercises out of a trumpet book called the Arban book. So some guys just started calling him Arban behind his back. A lot of the guys gradually learned to like him, but some guys wanted to play tricks on him so that maybe he would quit. But Carl was rustic and countrified and he used those Pa Kettle expressions like 'By Granny' and 'gettin' a lickin'.' He was a Rube and very naive at that time. He was like Lum and Abner too, charming, and you couldn't help yourself but like him and gradually he won us over. But not before he was conned into thinking that the police and an angry father were on his trail for compromising a certain young lady's virtue.[25]

When Severinsen came back to Portland, he began playing with the Walter Bridges big band and jamming at the Coop and the Acme, where one of the trumpet players in the Bridges band remembers him as an excellent lead but not into some of the modern things that

Bobby Bradford and Evans Porter were doing. In 1947 he joined the George Bruns KOIN radio band. On one side of him sat Don Kinch and on the other Don Proctor from the Clover Club. "He wasn't a character in those days," says Proctor. "He was shy and retiring, not like you see on TV with Johnny Carson. He was here from about 1945 to '47. Of course he had unheard-of power in those days. He could actually rattle the light fixtures. That person that you see on TV isn't all that much of a fake. Doc Severinsen really was a hip hick."[26]

Doc Severinsen's role as an educator must give him the most satisfaction, because for four decades he has performed in hundreds of high schools and colleges. When he was at the University of Portland in 1964, he was on a mission to upgrade the level of music in America. To a large gathering of would-be brass players between the ages of seventeen and twenty-two, Severinsen put on a dazzling display of versatility— symphonic pieces, swing numbers, show tunes. He wasn't just grandstanding. His point was that, even in the mid-sixties, you don't just stomp your feet and go into "The Saints Go Marching In." And then he put down his trumpet and went into a fifteen-minute down-home sermon. He told them he did clinics because of the inspiration he got from the great Tommy Dorsey when they were playing at the Paramount Theater. Because of a contest he won, he was asked to come into Portland to play with the Tommy Dorsey band. He was fourteen, and after it was over, guys like Ziggy Elman took him aside and helped

him out. He never forgot that. So this is his way of passing some of the most important pointers along. "First," says Severinsen, "learn to play everything, from polkas to classics, and start with classical music first because it makes everything else easier. Then work on your tone." Severinsen talked about the relationship between language and music, notes and words, choruses and paragraphs, about how to build a solo. Then, he said, if they decided on jazz, get your roots deep. "Don't just start listening to the avant garde like Don Cherry or even Miles Davis. Go way back. Go back to the recordings of Freddie Keppard, Dizzy Gillespie, Louis Armstrong, Rex Stewart." And then he ended with an urgent plea to upgrade the music in America by setting high standards, standards that they themselves can pass on.[27]

CHAPTER 16

Paul's Paradise

Paul's Paradise came into its own when the south end of Williams Avenue was surrendering to the power of freeways. It was a few doors down from the corner of Russell and Williams. It is all part of the Emanuel Hospital landscape now, but from 1955 through '57 it was the busiest corner on the Eastside. "Like NW 23rd on Saturday," says James Benton, "where all the pretty girls and all the pretty guys would hang out—at Porter's, Citizen's, or at Paul's." Paul was Paul Stewart. He owned the club and liked the idea of a workingman's Chicken Coop, with a louder, less restrained audience, as in wide silk ties,

two-toned shoes, pinky rings, and a Dobbs lid from Lew's men's shop across the street. There was rhythm and blues at Paul's, something you wouldn't find at the Chicken Coop. The bop was harder too. Art Blakey, Clifford Brown, and Horace Silver's "Opus de Funk" were the standards to strive for.[1]

Paul's was the scene of some unforgettable summit meetings, nights never recorded but fresh in the memories of those who were there. The competition was fierce. You might find yourself in the middle of two world-class sidemen from the Count Basie band, as Al Johnson did in 1953, one night after the

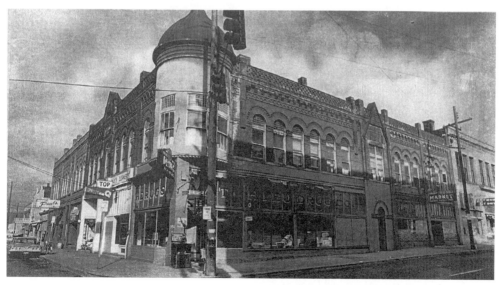

Paul's Paradise is on the left of the photograph, where the car is parked (courtesy of Oregon Historical Society, negative # 1691)

Basie band had finished a dance job. "Frank Foster and Frank Wess and me in the middle," says Johnson, "and do you know what they made me do? They made me start 'Perdido' all by myself and I kept thinking 'What am I doing here, I'm just getting started.' "[2]

The former music columnist John Wendeborn survived Paul's baptism of fire in the days when he was playing his single-trigger trombone. He went home and wrote a story called "The Badge" about how it is to be the only white musician in an all-night, all-Black cutting session. When Wendeborn arrived, waiting for him at the top of a ladder that led to a small loft, were Evans Porter, Bobby Bradford, and Wendeborn's sparring partner, Cleve Williams. Wendeborn writes,

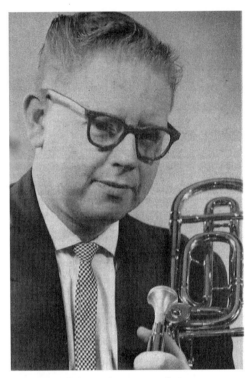

John Wendeborn (courtesy of Margaret Havlicek and Phil Hunt)

Cleve Williams had little time for anything but jazz. He was the kingpin trombone player on the Avenue. Three horns went into a familiar Bird-penned blues for two trombones and a trumpet. When Evans Porter snapped off a medium funk tempo, the drummer crescendoed a stick roll on his snare, and the white boy [Wendeborn] stepped up to the mike and out came a torrent of notes, the slide working smoothly as his solo gained in emotion. The crowd erupted in cheers as Cleve stepped to the microphone and then Bradford and then Evans Porter followed, taking the tune into uncharted territory with devastating chords and looping right-hand lines and then it was over. The white boy moved down the ladder to find a guy holding his

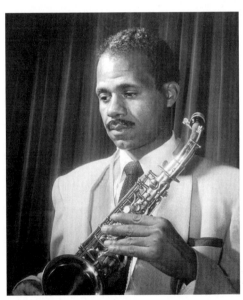

Roscoe Weathers (courtesy of James Benton)

trombone case for him. "Can I carry it for you?" he asked.

The ultimate compliment. The badge.[3]

Wendeborn hung up his horn in the sixties to become a jazz journalist and jazz promoter, going all the way back to the time he brought Miles Davis to the old Oriental Theater to the present with his Instrumental and Vocal Madness concerts. His biggest contribution, however, was as a music critic for *The Oregonian* from 1971 to 1985. Wendeborn was one of the few reviewers that musicians could rely on for a thoughtful and knowledgeable assessment of their performance.

Another piano player at Paul's was Randy Bogard, a gangly unkempt self-described cross between Bud Powell's jabbing left hand and Horace Silver's trumpet-styled right. Bogard played the piano face down, his nose hovering inches above the keyboard as if he were nodding off like Bill Evans. He was death on rock and roll even beyond the usual contempt among believers in Parker and Gillespie. Just the mention of it and he would be reaching for a revolver.

The legends of Jackson Street in Seattle, that city's version of Williams Avenue, liked to play at Paul's. Altoist Roscoe Weathers came down to Portland and became a temporary resident, joining Les Williams, Pony Poindexter, and George Lawson at a time when there might have been more talent on that instrument than on any other, with the possible exception of piano. Seattle's jazz historian, Paul de Barros, says that Weathers "had blown away everybody in Seattle." He did the same in Portland the way Sonny Criss had done in 1947. Criss and Weathers are both from Memphis, Tennessee, where Hank O'Day was the big man on saxophone. Both have a vibrettoless, panic-stricken sound close to Charlie Parker, to whom they were devoted, convinced that his music was the highest expression of American art.

Ken Boas, a Seattle piano player who played at Paul's Paradise with Roscoe Weathers, recalls standing next to Weathers in a nightclub listening to "Scrapple from the Apple" by Parker on a jukebox. "I'll never forget. Roscoe turned to me and he had tears coming down his eyes. I said 'What's the matter?' He said, 'You don't understand. Those guys, Wardell and Bird, it's just like they are praying.' "[4] Weathers made an album under his own name; however he is in better form on an Andex LP done in the late fifties called *Stringin' Along*.

Seattle's Jabbo Ward had been coming to Portland since 1945, when he was a member of the Al Pierre group at the Dude Ranch. His tenor battles with Sherman Thomas at Paul's and his baritone saxophone work with colleague Billy Tolles at the Tropics helped to increase his popularity and his impact on other Portland saxophonists.

Floyd Standifer is not the only outstanding trumpet player from the Emerald City. Neal Friel is another. "Friel is the blowin'est cat I ever stood next to," proclaims the normally taciturn Bradford. "He was a compulsive off-the-wall character out of a jazz novel," says Paul de Barros. "At fifteen, he used to run home every day to hear Sonny Berman

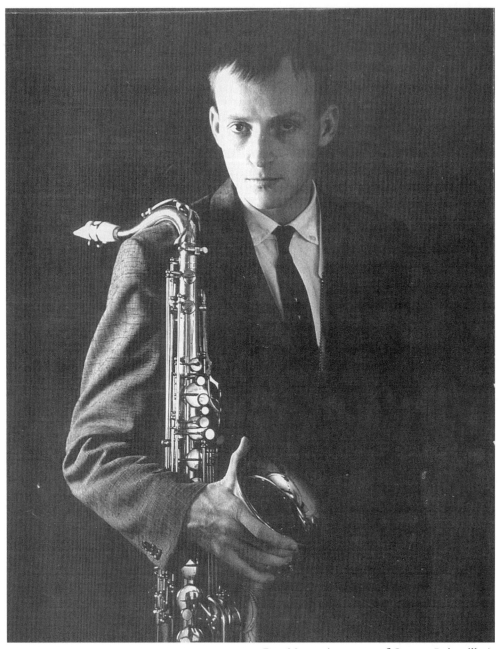

Dan Mason (courtesy of George Reinmiller)

play Woody Herman's 'Sidewalks of Cuba' on his record player."[5] Coincidentally, it was with Woody Herman that Neal Friel recorded his best-known solo.

On weekends there would be a long line of drummers waiting to sit in at Paul's, except when Seattle's Buzzy Bridgeford was in town. Then the locals, some of them, like Mel Brown and John Sumner, still in high school, came to watch, listen, and learn. Ray Spaulding was among them. "Buzzy's appearances would be like an event, man. All the drummers in town would get on the phone to tell each other to be at Paul's because he'd usually be there just one night. He always looked ill when he was there. Larry McKenna and a lot of other drummers came under his spell and we would just sit there by the hour taking in every move."[6]

When Don Manning of KBOO was beginning drums, Buzzy Bridgeford was his informal teacher and model. "He was a little guy, very frail, always looking down at the floor like some Kerouac character," says Manning.[7] Drummers noticed the sound of his cymbal, a sound they compared to drummer Art Mardigan of Woody Herman's band. Bridgeford is the drummer with Randy Brooks on a Decca recording, "Tippin' In," and later made a record with Tacoma, Washington's, famous Corky Corcoran.

When he wasn't on the road with Erroll Garner, Seattle's bassist Wyatt Reuther was a frequent visitor to Paul's bandstand, sharing the stage with Gordon Jackson, Charles and Mary Lockridge, and another bass player hardly

anyone remembers, Dick Kniss. Kniss grew up in the mid-fifties in Portland, living with his grandparents just off SE 12th and Stark. He started off as a guitar player but was persuaded by the influential Randy Bogard to switch to bass. Bogard showed him the positions on the string bass but never taught him to read music. Later Kniss found a German bass and began showing up at Paul's or at Sylvia's on Vancouver, his favorite place to play with his favorite quintet of Randy Bogard, Lee Rockey, George Lawson, and Dan Mason. Mason remembers that they used to turn down jobs so that they could all play together. They would end up playing from eight at night until six in the morning and then go off to the Coop for more. A cement contractor by day, Mason was part of the crew that bulldozed Sylvia's to make way for the freeway.

Kniss moved to Troy, New York, not long afterwards and eventually won an audition with the great Woody Herman band, until the band got to Dubuque on its road trip when Kniss found out that Herman had two books of arrangements, a jazz book that Kniss had memorized, and the easy-listening dance arrangements, most of which he would have to sight read. Two numbers into the program Woody Herman gave him that look that band leaders give when there is an impending disaster. And that was his short career with Woody Herman.[8]

Kniss worked on his reading and finally landed a job with the Don Friedman trio of the early sixties. They made some records for Riverside. The

best one is *Dreams and Explorations*,
with guitar player Attila Zoller. Former
Portlander Dick Berk is on drums. Like so
many, Kniss was taken by the
revolutionary bass style of Scott LeFaro.
He played with Toshiko Akiyoshi's trio
for a short time and then with the Pepper
Adams and Donald Byrd quintet at the
famous Half Note in New York City. Later
he joined John Denver and finally Peter,
Paul, and Mary, and can be heard on
many of their albums.

CHAPTER 17

The Playhouse Theater

McClendon's Rhythm Room was the most popular jazz spot on the eastside in 1953. On the west side of the river it was the Playhouse at 1117 SW Morrison, where the light rail turnaround is today. Guitarist Scotty Mills played there when her picture was on the front page of *Down Beat.* The great tenor saxophonist Dick Knight worked there for a while. What most people remember about the Playhouse happened in the beginning of November 1953 when Charlie Parker arrived with an all-star quintet. He was featuring the latest sensation, Chet Baker, an angel-faced trumpeter who was winning poll after poll, much of it based on his recording of "My Funny Valentine" with the Gerry Mulligan quartet. The winter of '53 was a low point in Chet Baker's health. He told Ted Hallock in an interview that night that he was giving up the trumpet because he was losing his teeth, a condition that affected all the members of his family.[1] His plan was to play piano for a couple of years and then give up jazz altogether. He found the right dentist, evidently, because 1954 and 1955 were better years for him.

When a young drummer named Ray Spaulding heard that Chet Baker and Charlie Parker and his favorite drummer, Shelly Manne, would be in town, he was the first in line to buy tickets.

Gene Norman was promoting the concert and he tried to sell the show separately but it didn't work because the attendance was kind of low. I remember the emcee, I won't mention his name, a disc jockey, got so depressed because of the turnout, that he got plastered and forgot to introduce Charlie Parker for the second concert. I was one of the people backstage who, with some other musicians, actually had to push Bird out on the stage, and, man, he played the best set I ever heard in my life. It was music that changes your whole way of thinking about music. When Chet and Bird were trading fours on "Cool Blues," I think it was, the octave key on Bird's horn went out on him. Anyway he came backstage and someone found a rubber band from one of Wally Heider's friends who happened to be taping the concert that night. It worked out fine and as Bird was coming back on stage he passes me and says, "Chet is really playing tonight, isn't he?"

The first concert that night was also inspiring. It was the Dave Brubeck quartet with the mighty Paul Desmond. They were doing tours of college campuses and becoming popular with students. Before coming here they made an album back at Oberlin College in Ohio that is still my favorite album after all these years. Well, that same band was at the Playhouse playing the first concert before Bird and Chet came on. It was Paul Desmond, Dave Brubeck, Ron Crotty, and Lloyd Davis. They were so basic compared to today. Lloyd Davis was a classically trained San Francisco symphonic percussionist. He only had a bass drum, a snare drum, a ride cymbal, and a high hat, yet the rhythm was so tight and the time was so right because he and Crotty played together for such a long time. He just played beautiful time in the background. You have to listen to that album to see what I mean. Anyway, I ran into Davis a few years ago after that in San Francisco. He had taken a day job and wasn't even playing. I told him how sorry I was about that and that his playing was inspiring to me that night in Portland and to the other drummers there. All he said was "Well, that's the way it goes."[2]

CHAPTER 18

The Olympic Room

The Olympic Room was the Avenue's last spark. It was located way out on North Vancouver and Fremont, about one mile from the corner of Williams Avenue and Cherry Court, the Avenue's original epicenter. Drinking was the priority at the Olympic Room. Music, as good as it was, came in second. In its prime, the room had some of the same acts as Paul's Paradise, including guitarist Al Mitchell, saxophonists Huey Lewis and Jimmy McCowan, and a trio of fine drummers named Johnny Cleveland, Malcolm Keyes, and a newcomer out of Detroit, Lawrence Williams. The house band was Basie Day and the Three Aces starring the Waltons—Cecil, Milt, and Teko—and their 7-on-the-Richter-scale version of "Caravan." Before coming to Portland with the Buddy Banks band in 1945, Basie Day had had a successful career accompanying Hollywood nightclub sensation, Hadda Brooks. He is on most of her early recordings.

"Basie Day was the Clown Prince of the Avenue. On Halloween and other holidays, he would dress up in drag," says Julian Henson, who played with him at the Olympic Room. "He would just fall over with delight every time he saw you in the street, like you were his dearest companion in the whole world. He died on the bandstand, the bass still in his

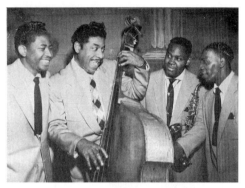

Left to right: Cecil Walton, Basie Day, Milt Walton, Harry Kenny (courtesy of Margaret Havlicek and Phil Hunt)

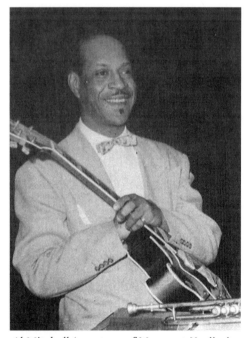

Al Mitchell (courtesy of Margaret Havlicek and Phil Hunt)

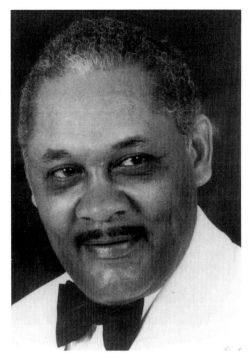

Sir Malcolm Keyes (courtesy of James Benton)

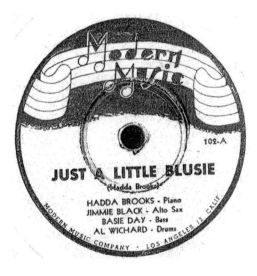

hands. The rest of the guys thought he was just putting us on like he always did, so that we didn't even call an ambulance until it was too late."[1]

By 1958, the Avenue was drying up faster than wet cement: urban renewal, Interstate 5, television, a change in popular music tastes from Ralph Martieri to Elvis Presley, the demise of ballrooms and big bands coming through all contributed. There was a change in the way people traveled, too, making it possible to fly over Portland. In the age of the steam engine and before the popularity of the airplane, Portland was a halfway stop for every vaudeville act, minstrel show, big band, and any other performing group using jazz musicians. If, for instance, the famous Duke Ellington played San Francisco and Seattle, he would have stopped in Eugene and Portland. There was a change in the Avenue's climate as well, resulting from a national vice probe focusing on Portland racketeer Jim Elkins and implicating associates such as Tom Johnson and his activities.

"None of the above would really matter," says Bill Hilliard, former editor of *The Oregonian*. "When the Exclusion Act was passed, lifting the red-lining practice of real estate agents and enabling Blacks and other minorities to live anywhere they wanted, Tom Johnson knew the handwriting was on the wall. If Black people could live anywhere legally, it would break up his principality. Businesses would move away and people would scatter."[2]

CHAPTER 19

The Cotton Club

Williams Avenue had an encore at the Cotton Club on Vancouver Avenue. That was in 1963 when Paul Knauls, an enterprising, sartorial young man from Spokane took over the "about to go under" nightclub. The Cotton Club was a less formal mid-sixties version of the Dude Ranch and an inevitable destination for Joe Louis, Sammy Davis, Jr., Big Mama Thornton, and other Black celebrities. As Knauls used to say, "If you didn't get to the Cotton Club, you didn't get to Portland." He put together a chittlin' vaudeville show that *The Oregonian* said "could not draw more people if he were to give ten dollars away after each number." As in the days of the Dude, jazz was just part of a line-up, sharing the stage with comics, exotic dancers, and female impersonators. Soul and rhythm and blues had replaced jump and boogie-woogie, and the tenor saxophone joined the Hammond organ and drums as the small combo of choice. Billy Larkin and the Delegates substituted the guitar for the saxophone and became an overwhelming success at the Cotton Club, with a number of record albums to their credit. Warren Bracken, Gene Diamond, Les and Cleve Williams, Bobby Bradford, and others continued to perform until business took a dramatic nosedive in 1968.[1]

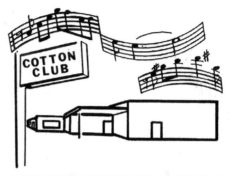

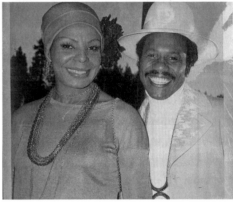

Paul Knauls and his wife Geneva in the 1970s (photograph and drawing above courtesy of Paul Knauls)

Knauls knows why:

There were riots everywhere. There were riots in Portland, too, after the deaths of Dr. King and RFK. It was a terrible time. Whites stopped coming up here. It was hard for them to come to this side of town since they were coming from Beaverton and Southwest Portland. The riots ended it. Then when Emanuel Hospital came in, that contributed to the demise. Doug Baker of the Oregon Journal *used to come to the club and write about it in the paper, and the next night the whites would come pouring in. Whites would come on Tuesday, Wednesday, and Thursday. Blacks would show up on Friday, Saturday, and Sunday. The place was going, I mean really going. At the end of the night, I would always say, "Thank you very much for coming to the Cotton Club, the only club on the West Coast with wall-to-wall soul." I would say "wall" and the rest of the crowd would say "to-wall soul" and then everybody would get up to leave.*[2]

Afterword

BY LYNN DARROCH

Of course the story goes on.

After the dust from the bulldozers had settled along Williams Avenue, after the clubs that had sustained Portland's golden age were replaced by freeway ramps and Emanuel Hospital, the story of jazz went on. After the mid-sixties, when the Black community was fragmented by physical and social change, the story went on.

Quietly at first, though.

In the late sixties, there wasn't as much jazz in town as there had been, and the scene was slow to rebuild. In fact, the story of the post-Williams Avenue era in Portland doesn't really start to take off until 1973, when Mel Brown, who had cut his teeth along the Avenue, came back to town, the Jazz de Opus began presenting live shows, and a jazz renaissance got underway that culminated in the boom of the eighties.

"There was no jazz here then," Brown recalls of his homecoming. "I couldn't even find a jam session. So I talked to George Fracasso at the Prima Donna, and Friday of the week we started there was already a line around the place." Though he exaggerated the music's plight somewhat, Brown was right about his appeal: thirty years later, he continues to be one of the city's biggest jazz attractions. More than any other single figure, Brown, who was born in 1944, best represents the story of post-Williams Avenue jazz in Portland.

While he was still in high school, he began to play professionally and attend jam sessions in the community. "At that time," he recalls, "Bobby Bradford and Cleve Williams would wait for me after school, and they'd show me how to set up certain figures with the Walter Bridges big band. Later, Julian Henson probably taught me all of the basics about what's happening musically. Omar Yeoman brought me along, too. During that time, that kind of teaching of

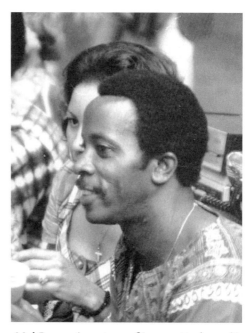

Mel Brown (courtesy of Joanne Hasbrouck)

younger musicians was what everybody did," he adds, "because they were helped that way themselves."

Brown attended Portland State University and played with Billy Larkin and the Delegates, one of the Avenue's premier organ trios, with whom he made his first album. Soon after, he went on tour with Earl Grant, where he was recruited for a job with Martha and the Vandellas. That began his eight-year association with Motown, when he toured and recorded with the Temptations and the Supremes.

Then Brown decided to come home, where the scene had changed.

Though the music had indeed fallen on hard times everywhere and had nearly dried up in the Black community, there was still jazz in the city during the late sixties and early seventies. A few first-generation beboppers, such as Warren Bracken, continued to work and mentor younger musicians, including Native American saxophonist Jim Pepper. And there were new players coming to town, such as trumpeter and composer Thara Memory, who has served as a passionate educator for many of his thirty years here and currently directs an award-winning band at Beaverton's Arts and Communication Magnet Academy.

In the late sixties, some of the Avenue's jazz had moved east on what is today Martin Luther King Jr. Boulevard, to the Upstairs Lounge, where Ron Steen, Tom Grant, and Pepper performed while still in high school. Nationally touring acts that included Gene Ammons and organist Shirley Scott also played the club. Pianist Mary Field played the

Candlelight Lounge, the reincarnation of Sidney's on SW 5th, and singer/pianist Terri Spenser also led a popular group. Bassist Andre Garand, pianists Harry Gillgam and Dick Blake (aka Richard Applegate), and drummer Tom Albering were also active.

Saxophonist and composer Pepper also played Portland frequently during this period, though he had moved to New York in 1964. Of Kaw and Creek descent, his powerful style wedded Native American culture to jazz so effectively that he won a prominent place in Europe's post-bop scene before his death from lymphoma at age fifty in 1992. His best-known tune, "Witchi-Tai-To" (based on a healing chant of the peyote religion), which was also performed regularly by the Tom Grant band a decade later, reached the Top Ten on jazz charts in 1971. A challenging personality, Pepper was a pioneer of jazz-rock fusion and profoundly influenced several Portland players, including pianist Gordon Lee, who figured prominently in the Mel Brown sextet of the late eighties.

The scene remained small, but changes were brewing.

New jazz studies programs in colleges and universities in the early seventies injected vitality and added legitimacy to a music long associated with the underworld. Mt. Hood Community College, for instance, turned out a group of players who went on to become leading figures, including Steve Christofferson, Gary Hobbs, Phil Baker, and several years later, the bassist Ben Wolfe, who subsequently worked with

Wynton Marsalis and Diana Krall. Big bands such as Stan Kenton's soon came to depend on such programs to provide fresh horns, and many Portland players spent time in such groups before returning to town with skills sharpened.

Likewise, the founding of the Jazz Society of Oregon in 1974, and the group's subsequent and continuing activities—which include a twenty-page monthly newsletter (currently produced by Wayne and M'Lou Thompson) as well as promotion of concerts and a scholarship program—helped support the growth of jazz. The group's early success in presenting jazz concerts demonstrated to club owners that an audience did exist. And that was crucial, because nothing has yet replaced the steady nightclub gigs that are the music's life blood. The number of eating and drinking establishments willing to present live jazz continued to grow.

In 1976, the Jazz Quarry opened on SW Jefferson near 12th Avenue, and over the next eleven years became one of the most important venues in the city for a variety of styles: the New Orleans sounds of Stumptown; the bebop and ballads of the house band, the Eddie Wied trio; and a variety of nationally touring stars that included Herb Ellis, Red Holloway, and Mose Allison. It also hosted the Walter Bridges Big Band, a unit active until the former Williams Avenue bandleader's death in 1984.

Wied settled in Portland in 1970, after earning a master's degree in art and spending fifteen years accompanying Las Vegas show bands. He became known as "The Professor," however, as much for his teaching skills as for his mastery of the keyboard. The ease, intelligence, and fluidity of his sound capture the essence of modern jazz, and though he has recorded infrequently, Wied has been influential.

Stumptown, an extension of the Castle Jazz band, was led by Gary Peterson and trombonist Pat O'Neal and kept the New Orleans sound alive with performances at the Quarry and other locations during the eighties. Cornetist Jim Goodwin was prominent, as was clarinetist Jim Beatty, who led a popular New Orleans-style group.

The Hobbit, in its original location on SE 52nd Street, also began to feature live jazz in 1976 with a performance by bassist David Friesen and guitarist John Stowell. An intimate room in its first location, with leaded glass windows and ivy-covered exterior, the Hobbit became a more important venue for both local and touring musicians after its later move to a larger space on SE 39th Avenue.

Though Brown led a popular trio at the Hobbit in those years (sometimes featuring vocalist Shirley Nanette), the club's early success was also built on Friesen, who settled in Portland in 1969. Often on the road, he established a pattern of touring mixed with local club dates that continues to the present. With melodic scope and rich sound, Friesen, born in 1943, developed his career via associations with established players, including pianist Mal Waldron, saxophonist Joe Henderson, and flutist Paul Horn. Friesen toured the former Soviet Union in 1983 with Horn's quartet, the first group of Americans to play concerts open to the Soviet public since the 1920s.

Also on that historic trip (and on eight albums with the bassist) was John Stowell. Renowned among teachers and guitar enthusiasts for his innovative approach to harmony, Stowell (born in 1951) moved to the city in 1976, but like Friesen, the globe-trotting minstrel spends more than half the year outside Portland, playing in Europe, Latin America, and around the U.S. Still, when in town he's a regular at jam sessions and local clubs, and since the late nineties, he has led the city's annual Guitar Summit. Partnered with him several times has been guitarist Jerry Hahn, another immigrant with a storied past as a pioneer of jazz fusion.

During the mid-seventies, keyboard player and composer Jeff Lorber—one of the most successful jazz funk stars of the seventies and a power in Los Angeles studios today—found his voice and his confidence when he moved to town. "As soon as I got to Portland," he recalled in 1978, "I started getting a lot of encouragement from the musicians. I was getting work, and all of a sudden I was considered to be a well-respected piano player. I never really enjoyed that status in Boston."

By 1977, Lorber was sitting behind an electric keyboard at Ray's Helm, flanked by thumb-slapping bassist Lester McFarland and funk drummer Bruce Carter. Two years later, Kenny Gorelick (now Kenny G) joined on saxophone and Lorber's career took off.

The supportive nature of Portland's jazz scene, noted by Lorber and other immigrants, grew out of the golden years on Williams Avenue. And it retained that cooperative, small-town character even as jazz grew into a major cultural force in the city.

The 1970s produced a population increase in Portland comparable to the growth spurt of World War II. During those years, Portland's image as a leader of "Ecotopia"—a maverick, progressive region blessed with a magnificent natural environment and a vibrant central city— drew members of the arts community, among them jazz musicians and those likely to support them.

And they did. As a result, jazz began to appear in unusual places.

Portland Center for the Visual Arts, for instance, dedicated primarily to curating forward-looking visual arts shows, developed a jazz series that brought the likes of progressive musicians Archie Shepp, Max Roach, and Roscoe Mitchell to town from 1979 to 1985. Portland's avant-garde scene was also well-represented in the late seventies and into the early eighties as drummer and composer Dave Storrs and saxophonist-composer Rich Halley released several albums. Other experimental groups, such as Freebop, played the Kingston on West Burnside, where pianist Gordon Lee also led a post-bop trio.

For the most part, however, Portland remained a town primarily interested in what had been the Avenue's stock-in-trade: straight-ahead jazz. That's what the majority of musicians played and what the majority of clubs required.

Indeed, an audience was developing again, and the musicians came to them.

In April of 1975, for instance, Dizzy Gillespie, Terry Gibbs, Mongo Santamaria, Chick Corea, Billy Cobham, and Weather Report appeared in Portland. By comparison, that's more than have appeared in any single month (outside the festivals) in 2004. By 1979, twenty-five clubs were presenting live local jazz at least some days each week, and several others, including the Jazz de Opus, the Earth, and Euphoria, occasionally booked national acts such as the Pat Metheny Group and the Heath Brothers.

In 1978, the Jazz Society joined promoters Jim and Mary Brown to inaugurate the Otter Crest Jazz Weekend, a three-day version of what's come to be called "jazz parties," where some two dozen musicians spend a weekend performing for several hundred dedicated fans in a retreat or resort setting. Those concerts brought more nationally known players to the area and demonstrated that an audience for jazz existed outside the nightclubs.

Then, in 1979, the Washington Park Zoo (now the Oregon Zoo) initiated a series of summer concerts called "Your Zoo and All That Jazz" that presented primarily local players to crowds of as many as 3,500 people in a grassy amphitheater near the elephant house. Though the series changed its musical focus in the late 1980s, the years it presented jazz were important in building public awareness and support for the music. Jack McGowan, who got that series off the ground, would later promote the first Mt. Hood Festival of Jazz.

Jazz was gaining respectability, and Portland was on the cusp of a new golden age, when, as guitarist Dan Balmer put it, "Musicians called Portland the place where jazz players own houses."

Despite the recession that slowed the state's economy in the early 1980s, a jazz boom accompanied it. The number of celebrated artists of all styles who played Portland was increasing, but what led Portland to be called "Kansas City on the Willamette" was primarily the nightclub activity—over forty clubs presenting live jazz weekly by 1981, supporting over one hundred twenty regularly active players. Chief among them at the time, in terms of influence and prestige (in addition to the Jazz Quarry, the Jazz de Opus, and the Hobbit, which were equally active) was Delevan's, a popular supper club located in a former firehouse on NW Glisan Street. Known for its food and ambience, Delevan's hosted national names such as Sonny Stitt and Eddie Harris. Accompanying many of these performers was the house trio: drummer Ron Steen, bassist Phil Baker, and pianist Peter Boe.

Baker went on to tour with Diana Ross, composed for and performed with Tom Grant, and is still one of the most active bassists in town; Boe followed bluesman Robert Cray onto the road. Steen, however, has remained in Portland for most of his career. Besides a tour with Harry Connick, Jr. and a stint in New York, he has dedicated himself to leading jam sessions that keep alive traditions he absorbed from players who once frequented the Avenue.

That fact helps account for his election to the Jazz Society of Oregon's Hall of Fame in 2002. But it's his musicianship that gives Steen authority. He has worked with Charles Lloyd, Joe Henderson, John Hammond, and Woody Shaw, has appeared on many local recordings, and performs nearly every night of the week.

During the boom years, two important outdoor summer festivals—both still alive in 2005—added variety and new listeners to Portland's jazz scene. In 1981, a group of volunteers were looking for an event to commemorate the construction of Cathedral Park under the St. Johns Bridge, and since Hank Galbraith—son of Howard Galbraith, who was known as "the mayor of St. Johns" and led the drive to build the park—was in the jazz business as owner of the Hobbit, the group started the Cathedral Park Jazz Festival in 1981. A people's festival with free admission, the three-day event continues to present national names in addition to a roster of local musicians.

The major-league Mt. Hood Festival of Jazz began in 1982 with a more ambitious agenda—three days of jazz by some of the greatest living players. The festival has gone through many changes: today it is held at the Gresham City Park ball field instead of the football stadium at Mt. Hood Community College where it began, for instance. Its biggest years were in the mid- to late eighties, when more than twenty thousand people attended during a weekend. The festival brought many performers to town who would not ordinarily appear here, and it also attracted many people unfamiliar with jazz who were out for fun in the sun with musical accompaniment. After the move in 2002, however, crowds have averaged less than three thousand for the revamped two-day event.

An additional sign of the increasing public profile of jazz was the start of the Museum After Hours weekly concert series in the Portland Art Museum in 1986, which initially featured local jazz exclusively and invited listeners into the exhibit halls to eat, drink, schmooze, and listen to music.

Perhaps the abundance of jazz in such nontraditional venues contributed to the problems nightclubs were experiencing. And some observers claimed that the summer festivals, which brought big-name artists to town for only a few days, were in part responsible for their decline at other times of the year. Nationally, the record business slumped in the early eighties as well. All of those conditions, in addition to increased liquor liability premiums, contributed to the loss of jazz clubs—between 1981 and 1984, the number of venues offering live jazz in Portland declined by nearly half. Cousins, a downtown club that had regularly hosted the Tom Grant band, closed in 1986. The Jazz Quarry closed in 1987. And other clubs cut back to duos instead of trios and quartets.

Nevertheless, some did thrive.

The Hobbit, for instance, presented a series of touring stars in the late eighties that included McCoy Tyner, Ray Brown, and Jim Hall. More important, however, was the development of the Mel Brown sextet at the club during those years.

Brown modeled his group after Art Blakey's Jazz Messengers. Brown's tight ensemble segued seamlessly from one hard bop tune to the next, creating a local following and winning the national Hennessy Jazz Search in 1989, when it opened the Playboy Jazz Festival and released *Gordon Bleu: The Mel Brown Sextet Plays the Music of Gordon Lee.*

The boom was also supported by four jazz radio stations, two of them full-time. All-jazz radio station KMHD-FM began broadcasts in 1984, and, with KOPB-FM (the Oregon Public Broadcasting network), community radio station KBOO-FM, and commercial broadcaster KKUL-AM, 170 hours a week of jazz aired on Portland radio during the mid-eighties. As was the case during Portland's golden age, dedicated disc jockeys communicated their knowledge of the music to listeners. At KMHD, for example, Bill Miller, Art Abrams, Bob Riddle, and Homer Clark created thoughtful, informative shows. At KOPB, George Fendel, Art Alexander, and Margaret's Aqua Lounge led the way. At KBOO, which played jazz when no others did, George Page, Gene Still, Don Manning, Jim Andrews, Garth Miller, Howard Cutler, and the urbane Charles de Greef were prominent. KKUL featured the return of Pat Patee, Ray Horn, and Ted Hallock, a Latin show by Cliff "Notes" Katanic, plus Rita Rega, Peggy Callomae, and Steve Brockway.

Another indication of the healthy state of jazz in the late eighties was the opening of Don Anderson's Birdland, Portland's first all-jazz record store. It was located across the street from the Multnomah County Central Library. Birdland lasted ten years.

Big bands continued to rehearse and perform, even though they have not been economically viable since the golden age, because big bands allow musicians to hone their reading and ensemble skills. Several of the most active of those groups during the eighties and nineties include The Woody Hite big band, the Mt. Hood Kicks band, the Art Abrams Swing Machine, Border Patrol, and the Carlton Jackson-Dave Mills big band. Drummer Chris Conrad also led a notable big band at a tavern called PC& S in the early eighties. Several other players have cut recent big band recordings of original work, including Gordon Lee and saxophonist Rob Scheps.

Don Mayer also bucked the trend to open the Village Jazz in Lake Oswego in 1985, where many national acts, including Mal Waldron and Barney Kessel, appeared. Also playing the Village Jazz was Charlie Rouse, the saxophonist for Thelonious Monk during his heyday; Rouse lived in the area until his death from cancer in 1988. But the nightclub market had become saturated, a trend that continued into the early nineties, when both the Hobbit and Remo's (the former Delevan's) closed. Many musicians found ways to survive and even prosper, though, as the economy of the nineties brought more opportunities.

Some of those opportunities were what musicians call "corporate gigs"— private parties sponsored by businesses. These usually pay better than nightclub work, and their number increased as the state's economy expanded. The big story of the nineties, however, was the rise of the Jazz de Opus as the hot spot for local jazz.

One of the groups that played regularly through the decade and built a following there was the duo of pianist and composer Steve Christofferson and vocalist Nancy King. They also appeared regularly at the RiverPlace Hotel on the Willamette, which also featured pianist Jessica Williams, who resided in Portland for a period in the nineties. Christofferson, who has several albums of his own as a leader, received co-billing on King's most significant album of the decade, *Straight Into Your Heart,* recorded with the Metropole Orchestra of The Netherlands.

King, born in 1940, has been considered the top jazz singer in the area ever since she emerged as the leader of a band at the University of Oregon that included Ralph Towner and Glen Moore, who went on to international stature as members of the group Oregon. Moore, who returned to Portland in the nineties, made a series of whimsical CDs with King singing lyrics by Moore's wife, Samantha. Moore, who teaches and tours most of the time, also occasionally plays in Portland clubs while in town. He has two solo CDs in addition to his work with Oregon and has played on contemporary classical music projects. Though King won the Talent Deserving Wider Recognition award in 1994 from *Down Beat* magazine, she, on the other hand, has never attained that kind of success.

During the same period, drummer Dick Berk, who had played with legends such as Billie Holiday, moved to the area

and remained active until he left for Las Vegas in 1996. Another drummer—Alan Jones, a Portland native who attended Berklee College of Music in Boston and worked in Europe and Canada before returning to town in the nineties— composed for and developed a hard-bop sextet that built an enthusiastic following at the Jazz de Opus. In fact, with the Leroy Vinnegar quartet and the trios of Dan Balmer and Don Alberts, the Opus had a cadre of regular groups that drew crowds enough to create a real scene at the Old Town club. Many of the listeners were under thirty years of age, a welcome turn for a music whose audience had been aging. The youth crowd also came out for Vinnegar—the beloved and respected master of the walking bass who appeared on hundreds of recordings during his years in L.A. and moved to Portland in 1986. Before he died in 1999 at age seventy-one, Vinnegar's impact was felt throughout the local scene, and Jones composed and recorded a CD titled *The Leroy Vinnegar Suite* in his honor.

Younger listeners did turn to jazz in the nineties, but many of them were drawn to the style known as smooth jazz. In Portland, the leader in that genre was singer and keyboard player Tom Grant, who developed his radio-friendly sound in local clubs as well as on the road. With guitarist Balmer, drummer Carlton Jackson, and bassist Jeff Leonard, Grant made a number of popular CDs before returning to the straight-ahead style after 1995; after all, he'd grown up on that music at his father's Madrona record shop, which served the Williams Avenue community in the forties and fifties. By 2000, the smooth jazz radio station that operated in town in the nineties had closed and the Smooth Jazz festivals that drew partying crowds in the summers were no more. But Grant has remained one of the city's biggest attractions and best-known musicians.

Another singer-pianist with an impressive discography who had a major impact on the local scene during the nineties was Dave Frishberg. He settled in Portland in 1986 but didn't develop a notable local presence until a three-year run at the downtown Heathman Hotel from 1991 to '94 with singer Rebecca Kilgore and a repertoire of jazz tunes from the thirties and forties. The Heathman has continued to offer piano jazz and occasional vocalists. Kilgore, who has recorded and toured with traditional jazz ensembles, got her start in the thirties-style swing band, Wholly Cats, led by cornetist Chris Tyle.

Since the seventies, there has always been some Latin jazz in Portland, and though Hispanics increased to more than 7 percent of Multnomah County's total population by 2004, they are not the primary audience. The leading Latin jazz band of the nineties was the Bobby Torres Ensemble, which mixed jazz, R&B and Latin influences. Few Latin jazz stars besides Poncho Sanchez visit Portland, and his appearances are almost all at summer festivals, including another new entry that began in the nineties, the Vancouver (Washington) Wine and Jazz Festival, which has also featured Cuban expatriate trumpeter Arturo Sandoval. Vibraphone player Rick McNutt led a

Latin group before he joined Tall Jazz (which has remained active and popular to the present), and on radio KBOO, Nick Gefroh and Molly Little have kept Latin sounds available.

The avant-garde found a local champion in the Creative Music Guild in the nineties, and through the organization's fundraising and publicity efforts, a series of European and American practitioners of innovative jazz have appeared in small local venues such as the Old Church downtown or the Community Music Center on the eastside.

Despite the caliber of musicians available and the many opportunities for listeners to hear them—usually in nightclubs with little or no cover charge—musicians continued to report that there was not sufficient work to support them. And the number of nationally touring players performing in Portland declined from its peak in the early eighties as well. Coupled with budget problems at the Mt. Hood Festival, on one hand, and the defunding of music programs in city public schools on the other, the scene's precarious foundation became clear.

The brightest moment in recent nightclub jazz came late in 1996, during a conversation between Mel Brown and Jimmy Makarounis about the organ trio sound of Billy Larkin and the Delegates. Their mutual delight in that style led the recently opened Jimmy Mak's to become an incubator for a new generation of jazz players attracted to the grooving sounds of funk jazz. Following Brown but seeking their own sound, bands such as

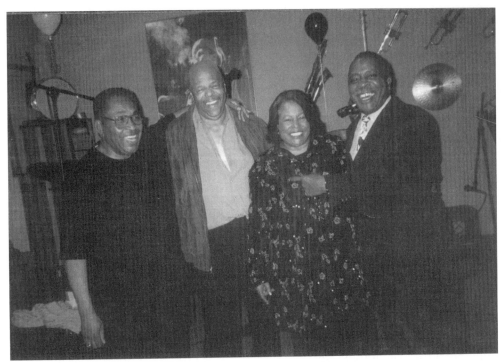

Left to right: Cleve Williams, James Benton, Marianne Mayfield, Mel Brown (courtesy of Cleve Williams)

the Jive Talkin' Robots and Groove Revelation played funk jazz from a Generation X point of view, reminding listeners that they come from rock as much as jazz. But Jimmy Mak's managed to attract both the young listener and fans who had heard music like this at the Cotton Club on Williams Avenue in the early sixties.

Though Brown provides a stylistic link to the Williams Avenue golden age, pianist and educator Darrell Grant has worked in other ways to maintain a connection to that heritage. A composer of funk jazz for his People's Music Project, a mainstream recording artist (his "Twilight Stories" was No. 3 on jazz radio charts in 1998), and a hard-bop improviser (his CD *Black Art* was named one of the Ten Best Jazz Albums of 1994

by the *New York Times*), Grant has made his mark on the community he adopted in 1996 by organizing a series of "Old Cats" concerts at Portland State University that put student musicians on the stand with Williams Avenue veterans.

In that atmosphere, a new group named the Original Cats emerged that featured Bobby Bradford, Cleve Williams, Bob Hernandez, and James Benton, all of whom had been active on the Avenue. Their drummer is often Mel Brown. One of the venues they play is the Blue Monk, which opened in 2002 with a mural of Brown and other local musicians in the stairwell and photos of jazz players on the walls. Another temporary resident who helped connect jazz to the community again was Grant's predecessor in the jazz studies department at PSU, pianist Andrew Hill. An iconoclastic composer, Hill was commissioned to write a piece commemorating the new Japanese American Historical Plaza on the city's waterfront.

Physical links to the past also remain. Downtown, the Brasserie Montmartre and the Benson Hotel Lobby Court Lounge continue to present live jazz, and in fact the Benson, where Jean Ronne has held the piano chair since 1974, is Portland's longest continuously running jazz venue.

A new annual festival got its start in 2004. The Portland Jazz Festival, whose artistic director, Bill Royston, formerly directed the Mt. Hood Jazz Festival, brought Wayne Shorter and other name artists to town in the winter for a hotel-based series of concerts downtown. Though the festival's first year was an artistic and financial success, the downturn in the economy after 2001 has affected the amount of jazz available in Portland. The most visible symbol of that downturn was the closing of the Jazz de Opus in 2003. When a stage for exotic dancers took the place of the city's most storied jazz club, it not only marked the end of an era but revealed how public perception of the music had changed since its days at the Dude Ranch, when "shake dancers" were a regular part of the entertainment.

In some ways, jazz in Portland has become respectable, has moved away from its association with vice and the underworld. But jazz is still rooted in the drive for freedom and self-expression, though it is often supported by universities and arts commissions and is used as entertainment at corporate parties. Most musicians still view it as an outsider's art, and jazz record sales don't even represent 5 percent of the national market. The number of Black musicians in town has declined markedly, and several attempts to present jazz in Portland's historically Black neighborhood (including Geneva's and Steen's Coffeehouse) have met with mixed results. But in other ways Portland's twenty-first-century jazz scene reflects the city's original golden age, and the spirit of the Avenue remains in the sounds of today.

The effort to capture forty years of jazz in Portland in one chapter means that not all who contributed can be mentioned. My apologies to all the musicians, club owners and managers, disc jockeys, and other supporters of the music who haven't been included here.

Lynn Darroch is a Portland writer and editor. His articles about jazz and culture often appear in The Oregonian.

What To Hear

Chapter 1. The Dude Ranch

Lionel Hampton, *Flying Home*, MCA (CD)

Buddy Banks, *Complete Recordings of 1945 to 1949*, Blue Moon (CD)

Floyd Standifer quartet, *How Do You Keep The Music Playing*, Night Flight (CD)

Jack McVea, *Complete Recordings Vol. III, 1946-1947*, Blue Moon (CD)

Lucky Thompson/Jimmy Hamilton (Earl Knight on piano), Fresh Sound (CD)

Chapter 2. The Castle Jazz Band

The Historic Castle Jazz Recordings 1947-1950 ("Floating Down the Green River" included), B and W Music (CD)

Don Kinch and the Conductors, Rex Recording (LP)

Chapter 3. Struttin' at the Golden West

Freddie Keppard, *The Complete Set 1923-1926*, Retrievel (CD)

Dink Johnson, *The Piano Player, Vol II, 1946-1948*, American Music (CD)

Chapter 4. The Acme

Lorraine Geller, *Memorial*, Fresh Sound (CD)

Dick Collins, Nat Pierce, *Nonet* (featuring Quen Anderson's writing), Fantasy (CD)

Herbie Mann, *Early Mann* (Lee Rockey and Keith Hodgson on drums and bass), Bethlehem Archives (CD)

Miles Davis, *At Last* (Lorraine Geller on piano), Original Jazz Classics (CD)

Leonard Feather Presents Cats vs. Chicks (Norma Carson and Bonnie Wetzel), MGM (LP)

Chapter 5. Lil' Sandy's

T-Bone Walker, Classic Rhythm and Blues (CD)

Billy Larkin, *Driftwood* (introducing Ralph Black), World Pacific (LP)

Chapter 6. Slaughter on Williams Avenue

Walter Benton/Julian Priester, *Out of This World*, Milestone (CD)

Jimmy Witherspoon, *Jay's Blues* (Cleve Williams and Roy Jackson appear), Charly Records (CD)

Chapter 7. Jumpin' at the Record Shop

Kenny Hing, *The Little King*, Quixotic Records (CD)

Sarah Vaughan, *Send in the Clowns* (with Kenny Hing and Count Basie), Pablo Records (CD)

Count Basie, *Farmer's Market Barbecue* (Kenny Hing spotlight), Original Jazz Classics (CD)

Chapter 8. Jumpin' at the Savoy

Sonny Criss, *Saturday Morning, Xanadu* (with Leroy Vinnegar) (LP)

Sonny Criss, *California Boppin'* (some tracks recorded at the Savoy with Wardell Gray and Al Killian), Fresh Sound (CD)

Eddie Wied, *In Italy*, Samjazz (CD)

Dick Blake, *How Deep Is the Ocean*, Pillar (CD)

Bob Crosby, *Accent on Swing* (Don Brassfield solos on a couple of tracks), Giants of Jazz (LP)

Luke Jones and Doctor Sausage, (Clarence Williams sings on four of the selections), Blue Moon (CD)

Wardell Gray and Dexter Gordon, *Jazz Concert West Coast*, Savoy (CD)

Percy Mayfield, Volume 2 (Roy Jackson can be heard on two cuts), Specialty (CD)

Big Jim Wynn, *Classic R & B 1947-1949* (CD)

Jean Ronne, *Isn't It Romantic* (with help from Scott Steed's bass, Lee Wuthenow's very cool tenor, and the artful brushwork of Neil Masson), Pillar (CD)

Chapter 9. McClendon's

Wardell Gray, *Live at the Haig '52*, Fresh Sound (CD)

George Shearing, Verve Jazz Masters (CD)

Oscar Peterson, *The Trio Set* (includes "Tenderly"), Verve Jazz Masters (CD)

Billy Eckstine, *Everything I Have Is Yours* (Warren Bracken is on four of the small group sessions), Savoy (CD)

Chapter 10. The Frat Hall

Jimmy Forrest, *Night Train*, Delmark (CD)

Slim Gaillard, *Slim's Jam*, Drive Archive (CD)

Marty Paich, *Moanin'* (includes Bill Hood's solo on "Warm Valley"), Discovery (CD)

Mary Lou Williams, *First Ladies of Jazz* (Dick Wilson small group gems), Savoy (CD)

Charlie Barnet, *Drop Me Off In Harlem* (Ernie Hood on one or two of the twenty selections), Decca (CD)

Hank Bagby, *Opus*, Protone (LP)

Chapter 11. DeLisa's and the Medley

Johnny Otis, *The Original Johnny Otis Show* (Mel Walker, Little Esther), Savoy (CD)

Erroll Garner, *Long Ago and Far Away* (includes "Laura"), Columbia (CD)

Chapter 12. The Chicken Coop

Sid Porter, *Gentle Giant*, Tiffica (still out there in used record shops) (LP)

Bob Crosby, *First Time* (Tommy Todd plays piano and wrote most of the arrangements) (LP)

Lionel Hampton, *Original Stardust Album* (Tommy Todd on piano), Decca (CD)

Stan Kenton, *Uncollected Stan Kenton (1944-1945)* (Englund's bass is upfront and palpitating on "St. Louis Blues"), Hindsight (LP)

Stan Kenton, *Innovations* (recorded live two nights before Portland appearance in February 1950), Flyright Records (CD)

Stan Kenton, *Festival of Modern Jazz* (recorded at Civic Auditorium in Portland in 1954), Status (CD)

Stan Kenton, *Kenton '76* (this album has many Mt. Hood Community College personnel including Dave Barduhn's sensational arrangements of "Send in the Clowns" and "Funny Valentine"), Creative World (LP)

Artie Shaw, *Indispensable Artie Shaw* (Ralph Rosenlund on many cuts), RCA Classics (CD)

Jim Beatty, *Live at Harvey's* (Harold Koster on piano), Vector Records (LP)

Chapter 13. McElroy's Ballroom

Dizzy Gillespie, *Pasadena Concert*, GNP (CD)

Johnny Hodges, *Used To Be Duke* (Coltrane as a sideman), Verve (CD)

Jimmie Lunceford, *Lunceford Special*, Columbia (CD)

Duke Ellington, *At McElroy's*, Laserlight (5 volume CD)

Tex Beneke, *On the Beam* (Norm Leyden arrangements), Magic (CD)

Erskine Hawkins, *Original Tuxedo Junction*, RCA/Bluebird (CD)

Joe Liggins, *The Shuffle Boogie King* (the complete "Honeydripper" plus much more), Proper (CD)

Tiny Bradshaw, *Walk the Mess*, Westside Records (CD)

Chapter 14. Uptown Ballroom

Woody Hite, *Sentimental Swing*, Medical Records (CD)

Boyd Raeburn, *Experiments in Big Band Jazz* (Milt Kleeb's "Boyd's Nest" in lineup), Musicraft (CD)

Chapter 15. Jantzen Beach

Les Brown, *Les Brown at Jantzen Beach*,
   Jazz Band (CD)
Woody Herman, *Jantzen Beach*, Status (CD)
Ken Baker, *Ben Pollack*, Jazum (LP)
Gene Krupa, *It's Up To You, Vol. 2*, Hep
   (CD)
Rod Levitt, *Dynamic Sound Patterns*,
   Riverside (CD)
Doc Severinsen, *Tonight Show*, Amherst
   (CD)

Les Brown, *Live at the Palladium*, Jazmine

(CD)

Chapter 16. Paul's Paradise

Woody Herman, *Concert for Herd* (Neil
   Freil is soloist on "The Horn and the
   Fish"), Verve (LP)
Don Friedman, *Dreams and Explorations*
   (Dick Kniss is prominent throughout),
   Riverside (CD)
Bob Keene, *Stringin' Along* (Roscoe
   Weathers gets this otherwise academic
   encounter off its feet with some fiery
   alto breaks), Andex (LP)

Chapter 17. The Playhouse Theater

Chet Baker/Charlie Parker, *Birth of Bebop* (a
   few tracks are from a concert done just
   days before their appearance at the
   Playhouse in November 1953), Stash
   (CD)

Chapter 18. The Olympic Room

Hadda Brooks (Basie Day heard
   throughout), Jukebox Lil (LP)

Chapter 19. The Cotton Club

Billy Larkin and the Delegates (Mel Brown
   on drums), Aura (LP)

Notes

Introduction
1. MacColl, E. Kimbark, *Growth of a City*

Chapter I
1. Ostransky, Leroy, *Jazz City*, preface
2. Interview with Bill McClendon, May 1994
3. Interview with James Benton, January 1995
4. Interview with Cleve Williams and Bobby Bradford, February 23, 1995
5. *People's Observer*, May 31,1945
6. Interview with Bernice Slaughter, June 1994
7. Interview with Richard Lachenmeier, owner of Multi-Craft Plastics, May 1997
8. Northwest Enterprise, June 6, 1945
9. *Life* magazine, July 11, 1938
10. Manley Maben, *Vanport*, p. 5
11. Interview with Bob "Sleepy" Williams, April 1996
12. *People's Observer*, November 22, 1945
13. Leonard Feather, *Down Beat* magazine, December 15, 1954
14. *People's Observer*, December 10, 1945
15. Telephone interview with Floyd Standifer, September 1994
16. Interview with Florence Mills, 1999
17. Telephone interview with Floyd Standifer, September 1994
18. Robert S. Gold, *Jazz Lexicon*, p. 172
19. Peter Clayton and Peter Gammond, *The Guinness Jazz Companion*, p. 41
20. Arnold Shaw, *Honkers and Shouters*, pp. 51-65
21. Stanley Dance, liner notes to *Jumpin' at the Savoy* (Decca)
22. Interview with Art Chaney, August 1985
23. Telephone interview with Ray Horn, February 1996
24. *Northwest Enterprise*, October 4, 1940
25. Liner notes, "Happy Home Blues" by Buddy Banks sextet (Official)

26. *People's Observer*, January 1946
27. Jack McVea, liner notes to "Open the Door Richard!" (Jukebox)
28. Interview with Art Bradford and his wife, August 1995
29. Red Callender and Elaine Cohen, *Unfinished Dream, The Musical World of Red Callender*, pp. 59, 193
30. *People's Observer*, July 20, 1945
31. Liner notes, *Central Avenue Breakdown, Vol II* (Onyx)
32. Interview with Clarence Williams, June 1996
33. The *Oregonian*, November 25,1933
34. Tom Stoddard, *Storyville*, Vol. 28, April, May 1970
35. Degen Pener, *The Swing Book*, p. 214

Chapter 2
1. Interview with Ron Weber, Herbert Jobelmann's son-in-law, April 1999
2. Conversation with Monte Ballou at Django Record Co., 1977
3. The *Oregonian*, May 12, 1979
4. James Collier, *The Making of Jazz*, pp. 280-91
5. *Willamette Week*, August 8, 1978
6. Interview with Don Kinch by Neville Eschen, March 1, 1995

Chapter 3
1. The Institute of Jazz Studies, Rutgers University, Goines, "Early Jazz Trumpeters," June 1972
2. The *Oregonian*, November 23, 1914
3. Liner notes from *The Legendary Freddie Keppard* (Smithsonian), 1979
4. Samuel B. Charters and Leonard Kunstadt, *Jazz, A History of the New York Scene*, chapter 4
5. Martin Williams, *Jazz Masters of New Orleans*, pp. 19-25

6. The Institute of Jazz Studies, Rutgers University, Onah Spencer, "Trumpeter Walked on Capone," 1941
7. *Downtowner*, December 4, 1999
8. Leonard Feather interview with Dink Johnson, 1950
9. Gunther Schuller, *Early Jazz, Its Roots and Musical Development*
10. Telephone interview with Floyd Levin, September 1998
11. *Down Beat* magazine, October 19, 1951
12. The *Oregon Journal*, December 1, 1954

Chapter 4
1. The *Oregonian*, February 18, 1949
2. Interview with Sleepy Williams, September 2, 1995
3. *Northwest Enterprise*, January 12, 1944, and October 10, 1945
4. Interview with Cleve Williams, February 23, 1995
5. Interview with Clarence Williams, June 1996
6. Interview with Dexter Gordon on *Dexter Gordon, American Classic* (Musician)
7. Leonard Feather, *Inside Jazz*, introduction
8. *Life* magazine, September 29, 1952, p. 67
9. Interview with Ed Beach, May 1996
10. Interview with Cleve Williams and Bobby Bradford, February 23, 1995
11. The *Oregonian*, September 29, 1985
12. Ibid.
13. Ibid.
14. Ibid.
15. Ibid.
16. Sally Placksin, *American Women in Jazz*, p. 32.
17. The *Oregonian,* September 29, 1985
18. Ibid.
19. Ibid.
20. Ibid.
21. *Down Beat*, January 25, 1952
22. Interview for *Willamette Week*, October 5, 1981
23. Interview with Nick Gefroh, April 2003

24. Interview with Carl Smith, April 2003
25. *Willamette Week*, October 5, 1981
26. Interview with Colleen Knight, July 1986
27. Interview with Ernie Hood, July 1984
28. Ibid.
29. Telephone interview with Norma Carson, Florida, July 1984
30. Sally Placksin, *American Women in Jazz,* pp. 166-67
31. *Down Beat*, April 6, 1951
32. Sally Placksin, *American Women in Jazz,* pp. 166-67
33. Interviews with Lee Rockey, August 1982 and April 1985
34. Ibid.
35. Telephone interview with Joy Rockey, March 2003
36. *People's Observer*, January 1946
37. Liner notes from *Saunders King* (LP, Blueboy)

Chapter 5
1. Liner notes from *Texas Music, Vol. I* (Rhino)
2. Interview with Frank Nudo, November 2004
3. Conversations with Ron Steen, May 2004
4. Interview with John Tanaka, July 1995

Chapter 6
1. Interview with James Benton, January 1995
2. Interview with Dick Bogle, August 1994
3. Arnold Shaw, *Honkers and Shouters*, p. 128
4. Interview with Bernice Slaughter, June 1994
5. Interviews with Cleve Williams, February 1995 and May 2003
6. Interview with Herb Amerson and Al Johnson, May 2001
7. Private tape from Robert Redfern collection
8. Interview with Cleve Williams and Bobby Bradford, February 1995
9. Interview with Ron Steen and Mel Brown, April 1997

10. *Down Beat Record Reviews, Vol. 6*
11. Interview with Bill Hilliard, September 1995

Chapter 7
1. Interview with Dale Harris, December 1974
2. Interview with James Benton, January 1995
3. *Life* magazine, 1938
4. Interview with Fay Gordly, March 1995
5. Telephone interview with Bill Haseltine, September 1995
6. Interview with Ted Hallock, February 2004
7. Interview with Eddie Wied, October 1994
8. Interview with Bernice Slaughter, June 1994
9. Marshall Sterns, *Jazz Dance*
10. Interview with Kenny Hing, January 31, 1982
11. Ibid.
12. Ibid.
13. Private tape from Robert Thompson collection
14. Liner notes from Count Basie's *Farmer's Market Barbecue* (Pablo)

Chapter 8
1. Sonny Clay, *Storyville* magazine, Volume 61, October/November 1975
2. Conversations with Gene Confer at the Fine Arts Building, 1978
3. Interview with Don Proctor, 1994
4. Interview with Eddie Wied, 1994
5. Interview with Ed Beach, January 1995
6. *Down Beat*, March 1951
7. Private tape from the collection of Robert Thompson
8. The *Oregonian*, November 4, 1984
9. Interview with Julian Henson, September 1994
10. Paul de Barros *Jackson Street After Hours*
11. Interview with Dale Harris, 1994

12. Conversations with Marianne Mayfield, June 1990
13. Private tape from the collection of Robert Redfern
14. Interview with Clarence Williams, March 1996
15. *People's Observer*, 1947
16. Liner notes from Jim Wynn, *Blow Wynn Blow* (Whiskey, Women and...Record Company, LP)
17. Institute of Jazz Studies (Rutgers University) file on Wardell Gray
18. Interview with Warren Bracken
19. Letter by John Chellun Holmes to Don Manning, 1965
20. Jack Kerouac, *On the Road*
21. *Melody Maker* magazine, 1954
22. Interview with Bernice Slaughter, June 1994
23. Telephone interview with Tim Kennedy, August 1994
24. Interview with Warren Bracken, August 1994
25. Interview with Dale Harris, May 1994
26. Telephone interview with Ray Horn, May 1994
27. Interview with Al Hickey, September 1995
28. Telephone interview with Don Schlitten, September 1995
29. *Down Beat* magazine, 1977
30. Ira Gitler, *Swing to Bop*
31. Telephone interview with Ray Horn, 1994
32. Interview with Dan Mason at Elmer's, 2000
33. Institute of Jazz Studies (Rutgers University) file on Al Killian
34. Radio interview with Teddy Edward on KKUL. 1988
35. Gunther Schuller, *The Swing Era*
36. Interview with Tim Kennedy
37. Interview with Warren Bracken, August 1994
38. *Down Beat* magazine blindfold test, 1967
39. Ross Russell, *The Sound*

Chapter 9

1. Interview with Bill McClendon, May 1994
2. Interview with Warren Bracken, August 1994
3. Ibid.
4. The *Oregonian*, February 16, 1996
5. The *Oregonian*, March 28, 1978
6. Telephone interview with Chuck Phillips, March 1995
7. Interview with Dick Bogle, August 1994
8. Letter from Velma French, June 1996
9. Interview with Chuck Phillips, March 1995
10. *Down Beat*, June 4, 1952
11. Interview with Cleve Williams, February 2002
12. Ted Hallock interview with Oscar Peterson, *Down Beat*, May 7, 1952
13. Interview with Al Johnson, May 1995
14. Interview with Bill McClendon, May 1994
15. Telephone interview with Ray Horn, 1995
16. Interview with Bill McClendon, May 1994
17. Ibid.
18. Telephone interview with Suzy Patterson, March 1993
19. Joe Uris, *Trouble in River City*, Doctoral Thesis, Portland State University
20. Telephone interview with Bill McClendon, July 1995
21. Interview with John Tanaka, July 1995
22. Telephone interview with Bill McClendon, July 1995

Chapter 10

1. *Northwest Enterprise*, October 28, 1930
2. Interview with Clarence Williams, June 1966
3. *Portland Challenger*, September 9 and December 23, 1952
4. Telephone interview with Ray Horn, February 1994
5. Interview with Dan Mason, February 2002
6. *Willamette Week* article on Buddy Morrow, June 22, 1982

7. Arnold Shaw, *The Street That Never Slept, New York's Fabled 52nd Street*, pp. 225-27
8. *Northwest Enterprise*, December 13, 1945
9. Albert McCarthy, *Big Band Jazz*, pp. 210-14
10. Sally Placksin, *American Women in Jazz*, pp. 90-93
11. Los Angeles *Times*, January 11, 1991 (archived at Institute of Jazz Studies, Rutgers University)
12. Interview with Cleve Williams, February 25, 1995
13. Peter Vacher, *Jazz Odyssey, The Autobiography of Joe Darensbourg*, pp. 74-76
14. Leonard Feather, *Jazz* magazine, Fall 1959, pp. 7-12
15. Paul de Barros, *Jackson Street After Hours*, pp. 39-40
16. Liner notes to *First Ladies of Jazz* (Savoy, LP)
17. Albert McCarthy, *Big Band Jazz*, pp. 111-12
18. Interview with Bill McClendon, May 1994
19. Interview with Art Chaney, August 1995
20. Interview with James Benton, January 1995
21. *Jazzscene*, 1979
22. Interview with Warren Bracken, August 1994
23. Interview with Sheldon Brooks, April 1995
24. Interview with Art Chaney, August 1995
25. Author's conversations with Keith Klein, Django Record Co., 1976
26. Interview with Art Chaney, August 1995
27. Private tape from the Robert Redfern collection
28. Oregon Public Broadcasting radio interview, August 1989
29. *Down Beat* magazine, "Caught in the Act," June 4, 1964
30. Interview with Ernie Hood, July 1984
31. Ibid.
32. Ibid.

33. Leonard Feather and Ira Gitler, *Encyclopedia of Jazz in the 1970s*, pp. 178-79

34. Interview with Ernie Hood, July 1984

Chapter 11

1. Interview with Bill Hilliard, 1995
2. *Down Beat*, June 6, 1952
3. Written interview with Dick Bogle, March 2000
4. *Down Beat*, May 21, 1952
5. *Down Beat*, August 10, 1951
6. Interview with Bill Hilliard, 1995

Chapter 12

1. Interview with Ray Horn, February 1994
2. Interview with Robert "Sleepy" Williams, September 2, 1995
3. Sid Porter radio program with John Salisbury and Nola Bogle, KXL, April 1970
4. *Oregon Journal*, June 3, 1976
5. KBOO program on Braley Brown, April1981
6. Private tape from the Robert Thompson collection
7. Interview with Ralph Rosenlund on OPB radio, August 1984
8. Oregon Public Broadcasting radio series on Tommy Todd, September 1986
9. Ibid.
10. Ibid.
11. Ibid.
12. Ibid.
13. *Down Beat* record review, Vol. 7, pp. 188-89
14. OPB radio series on Tommy Todd, September 1986
15. Ibid.
16. Ibid.
17. Interview with Gene Englund, August 1986
18. *Willamette Week* article on Stan Kenton, March 28, 1982
19. Whitney Balliett, *Sound of Surprise*, p. 11
20. The *Oregonian*, February 12, 1950

21. Carol Easton, *Straight Ahead, The Story of Stan Kenton,* pp. 145-46
22. *Willamette Week* article on Stan Kenton, March 28, 1978
23. Liner notes for *Stan Kenton's Birthday Album* (Creative World)
24. Conversations with Chris Tyle, February 2003
25. Conversations with Tom Wakeling, February 2003
26. Private tape from the Robert Thompson collection

Chapter 13

1. Conversations with Ernie Hood, July 1984
2. Booklet on the Swing Era, a *Time/Life* record series, vol. 6
3. Interview with Art Chaney, August 1995
4. *The Lens*, Washington High School newspaper, June 1925
5. William McClendon, *Straight Ahead: Essays,* p. 57
6. *Portland Challenger*, October 31, 1952
7. *Northwest Enterprise*, July 1947
8. Interview with Hank Wales, July 1982
9. Interview with Betty Kemp, March 1998
10. Telephone interview with Stanton Duke, Jr. in Oakland, 1998
11. Gunther Schuller, *The Swing Era*, pp. 392-402
12. *People's Observer*, July 27, 1949
13. *Northwest Enterprise*, February 6, 1940
14. Interview with Bill McClendon, May 1994
15. *Oregonian* article on Duke Ellington, May 25, 1974
16. *Down Beat* magazine, May 21, 1952
17. The *Oregonian*, May 25,1974
18. Interview with Ted Hallock, February 1995
19. *Northwest Enterprise*, August 18, 1943
20. Interview with Sheldon Brooks, September 1995
21. Interview with Hal Swafford, February 1998
22. *Northwest Enterprise*, April 4, 1941

23. Ralph Gleason, *Celebrating the Duke and Louis, Bessie, Bird, Carmen, Miles, Dizzy and Other Heroes*, pp. 63-72
24. *Northwest Enterprise*, February 8, 1948
25. Interview with Lee Rockey, April 1985
26. Liner notes from *Dark Town Strutters Ball* (Jukebox); and Arnold Shaw, *Honkers and Shouters*, pp. 54-55
27. Gunther Schuller, *The Swing Era*, p. 423

Chapter14
1. Interview with Ray Spurgeon, July 1996
2. Private tape from the Robert Thompson collection
3. Ray Spurgeon article in *Willamette Week*, August 11, 1981
4. Interview with Herbie Hall at Nordstom's, November 2002
5. Ted Hallock article in *Down Beat* magazine, July 1, 1951

Chapter 15
1. Interview with Sammy Amato, July 1982
2. Ibid.
3. Ibid.
4. Interview with Steve Brockway, April 2001
5. Carol Easton, *Straight Ahead*, pp. 64-65
6. Jantzen Beach dance band schedule
7. Interview with Cleve Williams, February 2002
8. Jantzen Beach dance schedule
9. Private tape from Robert Redfern collection
10. Interview with Dan Mason, February 2002
11. *Down Beat* record review, March 26, 1964
12. Ibid.
13. Rod Levitt special on OPB (four hours), September 1986
14. Ibid.
15. Ibid.
16. Ibid.
17. McCarthy, et al., *Jazz on Record*, p. 344
18. Interview with Dave Frishberg, September 2004

19. Telephone interview with Marty Wright, May 2003
20. Interview with Ted Hallock, February 1995
21. Interview with Sam Amato, July 1982
22. Interview with Les Brown at the Hilton Hotel, November 1993
23. Ibid.
24. Charlie Barnet, and Charley Dance, *Those Swinging Years*, p. 140
25. Interview with Don Manning, June 1994
26. Interview with Don Proctor, June 1994
27. Private tape from the collection of Robert Redfern

Chapter 16
1. Interview with James Benton, January 1995
2. Interview with Al Johnson, May 2001
3. John Wendeborn, Unpublished short story
4. Paul de Barros, *Jackson Street After Hours*, pp. 86-87
5. Ibid.
6. Interview with Ray Spaulding, November 1998
7. Paul de Barros, *Jackson Street After Hours*, p. 123
8. Interview with Dan Mason, February 2002

Chapter 17
1. *Melody Maker* magazine, Ted Hallock article, November 21, 1953
2. Interview with Ray Spaulding, December 1998

Chapter 18
1. Interview with Julian Henson, September 1994
2. Interview with Bill Hilliard, May 1994

Chapter 19
1. *The Cotton Club Revisited* booklet
2. Leslie Rosenberg's interview with Paul Knauls, May 2003

Bibliography

Balliett, Whitney. *The Sound of Surprise*. New York: E.P. Dutton and Company, 1959.

Barnet, Charlie, with Stanley Dance. *Those Swinging Years: The Autobiography of Charlie Barnet*. Baton Rouge: Louisiana State University Press, 1948. Reprint edition: Da Capo Press, 1992.

Bjorn, Lars, and Jim Gallert. *Before Motown, A History of Jazz in Detroit, 1920-1960*. Ann Arbor: University of Michigan Press, 2001.

Bogdanov, Vladimir, Chris Woodstra, and Stephen Thomas Erlewine. *All Music Guide to Jazz, 4th Edition*. San Francisco: Backbeat Books, 2002.

Callender, Red, and Elaine Cohen. *Unfinished Dream, the Musical World of Red Callender*. London: Quartet Books, 1985.

Charters, Samuel B., and Leonard Kunstadt. *Jazz: A History of the New York Scene*. Garden City, New York: Doubleday and Co., 1962.

Chilton, John. *Who's Who of Jazz, Storyville to Swing Street*. Philadelphia, Pennsylvania: Chilton Book Co., 1972. Reprint edition: Da Capo Press, 1985.

Clayton, Peter, and Peter Gammond. *The Guinness Jazz Companion*. Great Britain: Guinness Publishing Ltd., 1986. U.S. edition: Sterling Publishing, 1989.

Collier, James Lincoln. *The Making of Jazz, A Comprehensive History*. New York: Dell Publishing Co., 1978.

de Barros, Paul. *Jackson Street After Hours: The Roots of Jazz in Seattle*. Seattle, Washington: Sasquatch Books, 1993.

Delaunay, Charles. *New Hot Discography, The Standard Directory of Recorded Jazz*. New York: Criterion, 1948.

DeMarco, Gordon. *A Short History of Portland*. San Francisco: Lexikos, 1990.

Dixon, Robert, and John Godrich. *Recording the Blues*. New York: Stein and Day, 1970.

Down Beat's Jazz Record Reviews, Vol. I-VII. Chicago, Illinois: Maher Publications, 1963.

Driggs, Frank, and Harris Lewine. *Black Beauty, White Heat: A Pictorial History of Classic Jazz 1920-1950*. New York: William Morrow and Company, Inc., 1982.

Easton, Carol. *Straight Ahead, The Story of Stan Kenton*. New York: Da Capo Press, 1973.

Feather, Leonard. *The Encyclopedia of Jazz*. New York: Horizon Press, 1955.

Feather, Leonard. *Inside Jazz*. New York: Da Capo Press, 1977.

Feather, Leonard. *The New Edition of the Encyclopedia of Jazz*. New York: Bonanza Books, 1960.

Feather, Leonard, and Ira Gitler. *The Encyclopedia of Jazz in the 70s*. New York: Horizon Press, 1976.

Gioia, Ted. *West Coast Jazz*. New York: Oxford University Press, 1992.

Gitler, Ira. *Swing to Bop: An Oral History of the Transition in Jazz in the 1940s*. New York: Oxford University Press, 1985.

Gleason, Ralph J. *Celebrating the Duke and Louis, Bessie, Billie, Bird, Carmen, Miles, Dizzy and Other Heroes*. New York: Dell Publishing Co. 1975.

Gold, Robert. *Jazz Lexicon*. New York: Alfred Knopf, 1964.

Goldman, Eric F. *The Crucial Decade and After: America 1945-1960*. New York: Random House, 1956. Reprint edition: Vintage Books, 1960.

Goulden, Joseph C. *The Best Years 1945-1950*. New York: Atheneum, 1976.

Kerouac, Jack. *On The Road*. New York: The Viking Press, 1955. Reprint edition: Penguin Books, 1991.

Kinkle, Roger D. *The Complete Encyclopedia of Popular Music and Jazz, 1900-1950*, Volume 2 and Volume 3. New Rochelle, New York: Arlington House Publishers, 1974.

Lee, Bill. *Jazz Class, Jazz Dictionary*. Shattinger International Music Corp., 1979.

Lord, Tom. *The Jazz Discography, Volume II.* West Vancouver, BC: Lord, Music Reference Inc., 1995.

Maben, Manley. *Vanport.* Portland, Oregon: Oregon Historical Society Press, 1987.

McLagan, Elizabeth. *A Peculiar Paradise, A History of Blacks in Oregon, 1788-1940.* Portland, Oregon: The Georgian Press, 1980.

McCarthy, Albert J. *Big Band Jazz.* New York: Exeter Books, 1974.

McCarthy, Albert, Alan Morgan, Paul Oliver, and Max Harrison. *Jazz on Record, A Critical Guide to the First 50 Years: 1917-1967.* London: Hanover Books, 1974.

MacColl, E. Kimbark. *The Growth of a City: Power, and Politics in Portland, Oregon, 1915 to 1950.* Portland, Oregon: The Georgian Press.

McClendon, William H. *Straight Ahead: Essays on the Struggle of Blacks in America 1934-1994.* Oakland, California: The Black Scholar Press, 1995.

McCormack, Win, and Dick Pintarich. *Great Moments in Oregon History: A Collection of Articles from "Oregon Magazine."* Portland, Oregon: New Oregon Press, 1987.

Ostransky, Leroy. *Jazz City: The Impact of Our Cities on the Development of Jazz.* Englewood Cliffs, New Jersey: Prentice Hall, Inc. 1978.

Pener, Degen. *The Swing Book.* Boston, New York, London: Little Brown and Co.,1999.

Placksin, Sally. *American Women in Jazz, 1900 to the Present: Their Words, Lives, and Music.* New York: Wideview Books, 1982.

Prescott, Tracy K. *A Beat in Time: The Early History of Jazz in Portland, Oregon.* Corvallis, Oregon: thesis, Oregon State University.

Reisner, Robert George. *The Jazz Titans, Including "the Parlance of Hip."* Garden City, New York: Doubleday and Co., 1959.

Russell, Ross. *Bird Lives: The High Life and Hard Times of Charlie Parker.* New York: Charter House, 1973.

Russell, Ross. *The Sound.* New York: Macfadden Books, 1962.

Schuller, Gunther. *Early Jazz: Its Roots and Musical Development.* New York: Oxford University Press, 1968.

Schuller, Gunther. *The Swing Era: The Development of Jazz 1930-1945.* New York: Oxford University Press, 1989.

Shaw, Arnold. *Honkers and Shouters, The Golden Years of Rhythm and Blues.* New York: Macmillan Publishing Company, 1978.

Shaw, Arnold. *The Jazz Age: Popular Music in the Twenties.* New York: Oxford University Press, 1987.

Shaw, Arnold. *The Street That Never Slept: New York's Fabled 52nd Street.* New York: Coward, McCann and Geohagen, Inc., 1971. Reprint edition (as *52nd Street: The Street of Jazz*): Da Capo Books, 1977.

Stewart, Rex. *Jazz Masters of the Thirties.* New York: Da Capo Press, 1982.

Stratemann, Dr. Klaus. *Duke Ellington: Day by Day and Film by Film.* Copenhagen: Jazzmedia ApS, 1992.

Ulanov, Barry. *Handbook of Jazz.* New York: The Viking Press, 1960.

Ulanov, Barry. *A History of Jazz in America.* New York: The Viking Press, 1955.

Vacher, Peter. *Jazz Odyssey: The Autobiography of Joe Darensbourg.* Baton Rouge: Louisiana State University Press, 1987.

Walker, Leo. *The Big Band Almanac.* Pasadena, California: Ward Ritchie Press.

Walters, Howard J. Jr. *Jack Teagarden's Music, His Career and Recordings.* Stanhope, New Jersey: Walter C. Allen, 1960.

Williams, Martin. *Jazz Masters of New Orleans.* New York: The Macmillan Company, 1967. Reprint edition: Da Capo Press, 1979.

Index